Take good
heart!

~ your

Dee _____

May 2021

D1551403

# I Don't Want to

# Die Like This

## A Survivor's Guide to
## Thriving After a Heart Attack

DENISE CASTILLE

Printed in the United States of America

ISBN: 978-1-952756-19-1

For details email vyp.joantrandall@gmail.com

# Dedication

*This book is dedicated to my mom Shirley. Thank you for giving me the cup by the handle (usually filled with tea) and encouraging me to do any and everything I say I want to do, including writing this book. I value the insight and guidance you always provide me. I am who I am because of the unequivocal support and love you give me every day.*

# Table of Contents

# INTRODUCTION

D o you know anyone with heart problems? Maybe someone you love...or even yourself? In forty-eight days, I went from a "nothing is wrong with your heart" medical exam to 99% blockage and a full-blown heart attack! Like most people who trust a doctor, I wanted to believe them when they insisted, "Denise, there is no blockage or valve problems!" Yet the gradually increasing pain over the next several weeks told me there was something wrong. How would you feel if more than one doctor said your pain was just stress? Exercise more and eat healthier food? I was only forty-six years old on July 2, 2015 when I suddenly collapsed at work and probably should have died. This story of my life-changing experience and the critical information I share, often with humor, could certainly save a life...maybe yours.

Studies and statistics show that black women are undertreated when it comes to heart disease. We are not diagnosed at the same rate as other races. Forty-nine percent of

African-American women over the age of twenty have some type of heart disease like[1]:

» Clogged arteries

» Stroke

» High blood pressure

» Angina (chest pain)

This means nearly one in every two black women in the U.S. has heart disease. According to the American Heart Association (AHA), some of the biggest risk factors for heart disease tend to be more common in African Americans than in people of other races. For example, diabetes, high cholesterol, and obesity increase a person's risk of developing heart disease. And, all of these are issues that tend to be more common in African Americans. Genetics can also play a role in a person's risk level. According to the AHA, research suggests that a gene carried by many African Americans can make the body more sensitive to salt.[2]

-------------------.
[1] *"Heart Disease in Black Women: The Big Issue You Might Not Know About" (2018, February 12). Retrieved from https://bwhi.org/2018/02/12/heart-disease-black-women-big-issue-might-not-know*
[2] *"Heart Disease in African-American Women." Retrieved from https://goredforwomen.org/en/about-heart-disease-in-women/facts/heart-disease-in-african-american-women*

Maybe subconsciously that's why I chose Dr. Johnson as my first cardiologist. I thought because she looked like me, she would go the extra mile. She would be kinder, educate me, and encourage me to pass the knowledge on to others. When I didn't know anything about heart disease, I expected her medical guidance and knowledge. Instead, her lack of energy and interest in caring for me seemed intentional. Unfortunately, I would find other highly educated cardiologists who were also quick to move me in and out of the exam room, leaving me clueless about my health and feeling frustrated about what to do.

What I learned from my heart attack and subsequent treatment is it's important to be responsible to educate yourself, advocate for other opinions, and wisely take appropriate action. Heart disease is not a death sentence, and you will survive and even thrive if you take key steps along the way.

Every day people from all walks of life go through all manner of difficult experiences. Mine was heart disease by way of a massive heart attack and subsequent arrhythmia causing a dangerously low heart rate that led to a pacemaker implantation. Through it I discovered I am passionate about helping people and using my voice and teaching skills to share my story in a way that meets other heart attack thrivers where they are, have been, or might be headed. I'm hoping this book will at times make you laugh and say out loud "Me too." Other times I want you to get mad enough to do something different— maybe for yourself or someone else. I want this book to impress upon you the importance of regular checkups and to seek medical attention and second opinions if your body tells you there is reason to be concerned.

I am not a doctor or in the medical profession. Though there will be medical terminology, this is NOT a medical book. The stories and information are not a diagnosis. Every person on a heart journey is different from the next. This book is about my experience, my heart story. May you find insight and value from it, feel encouraged to help someone you know, and take good care of yourself.

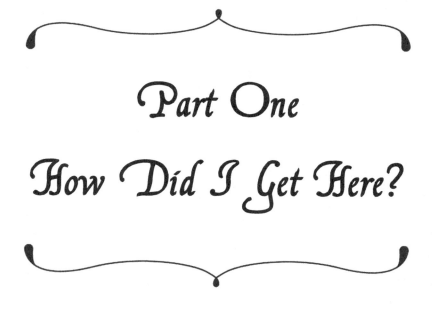

# Part One
# How Did I Get Here?

# CHAPTER ONE
# GRADUALLY THEN SUDDENLY

## *Recognizing Gradual Onset of Heart Disease*

*"How did you go bankrupt?"*
*"Two ways: gradually then suddenly."*
*—Ernest Hemingway's The Sun Also Rises*

I am a heart attack survivor. Never in my wildest dreams or nightmares did I ever expect to make that declaration.

Have you ever looked around and wondered, "How did I get here?" A burgeoning career or relationship, a couple of pounds here and there, or a symptom that may or may not be anything. Maybe no one could have diagnosed me with heart disease. Or perhaps the probability of a healthy forty-six-year-old having a heart attack was considerably low. Actually, the idea that something major happens in our lives out of nowhere is often a fallacy. Rarely does life bring us catastrophic results without some kind of warning. For many of us, including myself, we're not paying enough attention or taking action soon enough.

I agree with Steven Dennis and Seth Godin's idea that "Although unnoticeable, gradually eventually leads to suddenly. It builds momentum. It succumbs to the compound effect." Perhaps your gradually is getting out of debt with hard work and sacrifice or into debt with too many swipes of your credit card. My gradually were signs and symptoms I should have paid attention to. Your suddenly may be getting multiple credit card statements with a $0 balance. My suddenly was the widow-maker heart attack. But, how?

Like the character asks in *The Sun Also Rises*, how did I get here? Gradually then suddenly. It's 2015. Year after year, I ring in the new and out with the old. First and foremost, I always start by making the rounds to those whom I've named the *Big Five*: 1) gynecologist for my lady parts examination; 2) the embarrassing yet vital mammogram; 3) a date with my dentist; 4) the eye doctor to catch cataract and any other vision issues; and 5) my primary care physician for the all other free "well woman" appointment.

My amazing eye doctor, Dr. Thomas, is with Planx Eye Associates in Plano, Texas. When we moved to Frisco, about thirty minutes from Plano, I found an eye doctor close to my house. For no apparent reason, she wasn't going to prescribe colored contacts for me. I thought, "What the heck do you mean? Is there a medical reason I can't or shouldn't wear color contacts?" I had been wearing colored contacts for so long, sometimes I believed they were my natural eye color. As she continued to speak, I thought about what I would need to do to get a prescription for color contacts. I spoke up and asked, "Are the color contacts causing eye damage?" She casually said, "No." I said with confidence, "I prefer color contacts." She stared at me and wrote the prescription. I decided it was better to drive a little farther for excellent care, and I would be back with Planx Eye Associates. When I saw Dr. Thomas the next year, I couldn't tell he and the team enough about how sorry I was and said, "Please forgive me for leaving! I receive such good care from you." Lessons learned—speak up and choose excellence over convenience.

When we moved to Frisco, I found a primary care physician, Dr. Challa. I had a short list of must haves—I wanted a female doctor with an office not too far from the house, and she had to be in the network. Dr. Challa was a short lady with a heavy Indian accent. I loved that there was never a wait. In hindsight, maybe that should have been a characteristic to be concerned about instead of one to embrace.

My feet and ankles were swollen, and they had been for some time. They looked like matching balloons. We had tried a few home remedies. I increased my water intake, drinking eight to ten glasses of water a day. I would soak my feet nightly in Epsom salt. I cut out sodium...well, I reduced my sodium intake. My aunt recommended putting my feet up. Someone even suggested I walk to alleviate the swelling. All of the remedies were temporarily effective. Not one or a combination seemed to rid me completely of swollen feet.

They didn't hurt, but I wanted to be sure to mention them if Dr. Challa didn't say something first. It would be hard for her to miss them. I arrived for my appointment a little bit ahead of time. I was whisked to the exam room without delay. It seems they were a bit presumptuous as everything was set up to perform a pelvic exam. I quickly spurted out, "I have a gynecologist for that." The nurse obviously wasn't the person to converse with because she ignored me. When Dr. Challa came in, she explained that they were a one-stop shop, and I didn't need a separate gynecological appointment. I thought, "Well, I am already here" and agreed.

Dr. Challa checked all of my vitals. Looked in my ears, tapped my knees for a reflex, asked me to say "ahh" as she looked in my mouth. She had me follow her little pen light with my eyes. She checked my breasts for lumps and abnormalities. I asked her, "Since this is a one-stop shop, do I still need a mammogram?" She conceded, "Yes, you need to keep the appointment." I then endured the uncomfortable, "Put your feet in the stirrups and scoot your bottom more to the edge" exam.

Dr. Challa was washing her hands at the sink. I remembered to ask her about my feet. She dried her hands, came over, and felt my ankles. She took no time to deliberate or confer with her myriad of physician's books or colleagues and said as though she was about to tell the best kept secret, "It's because you're fat." There was a long silence. I was in disbelief that she said it, and this was the medical diagnosis I had tried to fix with so many remedies.

Dr. Challa never uttered a word that my swollen ankles and feet could be a sign of an underlying heart issue. She didn't point out when your heart isn't working well, blood flow slows and backs up in the veins in your legs, and it causes fluid to build up in your tissues. The truth of the matter is that I had been fat, to use her terminology, for some time but had never had swollen feet or ankles. Why didn't I point this out? She didn't stay for questions. She had said it and it was so. I didn't know it at the time, but that was my last visit to Dr. Challa.

In hindsight, there were so many red flags about this medical practice. When I had time to really think about my treatment, I realized I never had any blood work. What doctor doesn't do blood work?

If you work for someone, you are subject to performance reviews, right? Heck, even if you work for yourself your client will evaluate your performance. What is it about our medical professionals that we don't put them through performance reviews? I don't know about you but if I ever received a "needs improvement or doesn't meet expectations," I would be concerned for my job or business. For several years I allowed Dr. Challa to perform at a "needs improvement."

I am certainly culpable. There is no way that I should have walked away with a diagnosis of being fat as the reason for sudden swelling in my feet and ankles. Why were there no alarms that went off for either Dr. Challa or me? It would take a heart attack to do that.

### Denise's Words of Wisdom (WOW)

**Research:** Period. I know the Internet has made us all doctors in our own right. While we don't want to fall prey to self-diagnosis, we do want to be aware of what might be causing certain symptoms. If I had done any research, I would have been able to intelligently converse with my doctor and say, "All of a sudden my feet are swelling for no apparent reason. Is it possible this may be connected to my heart?" If in this scenario Dr. Challa replied, "No, it's not your heart, you're just fat," that would be all I needed to make a decision about her providing my care.

**Be Smart and Use Common Sense:** As I age it has been increasingly more difficult to lose weight. However, I had not gained any weight in the three years with Dr. Challa. What I am saying is this—it should have occurred to me that something wasn't adding up. If I was still overweight after three years, why would my feet start swelling now?

**Bloodwork:** Maybe my blood work wouldn't have shown anything. Maybe there would have been no signs for further investigation. But, just maybe it would have shown elevated cholesterol levels or something. Get blood work! If your doctor is not conducting blood work, then think about getting a new doctor. It should absolutely be part of a well-person exam.

**Stay in Your Lane:** You should stay in your lane and so should your doctor. Remember how Dr. Challa said they were a one-stop shop? Her specialty is general medicine. When it comes to a pelvic, my gynecologist should have done it. You may be thinking, "Okay, what does that have to do with your heart?" Directly? Nothing. But what if a doctor, with a different set of eyes, saw something or asked probing questions and got a different result?

**Self-Advocate:** Self-advocacy is when you speak up for yourself. You make decisions about your life, and in this case your health. The decisions you make come about after you gather information as a result of being curious. Ask questions.

Remember the not-so-good eye doctor? Her "why" for my not wearing colored contacts didn't supersede what I believed best for my eye health. And, quite frankly, it was a thoughtless and unprofessional answer. Just like the one Dr. Challa gave. I should have been equally deliberate about my physical health as I was about my eyes.

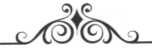

# Chapter Two

# Not One Bell or Whistle

## *Understanding Symptoms of Heart Disease*

*"Life's not always going to be bells and whistles."*
—*Gary Woodland*

When you look up chest pain on the Internet, it says, "Most people who experience chest pain immediately think they are having a heart attack." Nope—not me. There were no bells, whistles, or air horns for me. It was now March of 2015. My feet still resembled balloons. I was sporting open toe open heel flats like it was summer. I hadn't done any additional research on edema (swelling), so as far as I knew I would still have swollen feet until I lost weight.

One Saturday I was making the long drive to my tall African friend's place. This particular night we weren't going out. Kevin was cooking me a traditional authentic African meal. To make those thirty miles zip by, I always turned the music up. This time of the early evening the DJ was playing back-to-back good ole music. Like '90s old music and a little '80s mixed in for good measure. The music was so good to me that I had one hand on the steering wheel, and the other hand was my mic. I was having a blast and didn't care who saw me singing alone in the car.

I was about five miles away from Kevin's house, singing Atlantic Starr's "Secret Lover," when my mini concert was interrupted by *chest pain*. The feeling was completely foreign. I did what anybody experiencing a sharp, uncomfortable tightness and pressure would do—I turned the music down to concentrate and figure out what was happening. I'm talking a squeezing pain that wasn't letting up.

I put my fist mic away and said out loud, "Oh my goodness" and pressed my chest like pressing it would stop the pain. I assure you I hadn't lifted anything heavy, there had been no trauma to my heart, and it wasn't indigestion because I hadn't eaten anything. At this point I was much closer to his house than mine. I felt like stopping right then and there, but I decided to keep driving to his place.

Kevin was cooking stew with a red base and lots of fiery spices. I slowly and deliberately climbed the stairs to his apartment. I was winded when I reached the top of the stairs. I had climbed those stairs many times without being out of breath. The combination of being out of breath and the chest pain I'm sure shown all over my face. I knocked and walked in. I was fully prepared to pretend there was nothing wrong, but I couldn't. Without a word between us, Kevin knew that something was wrong. He came over and smothered his big arms around my short 5'4" body. "Please tell me what's wrong." I didn't want to spoil our evening and was evasive at first. "I'm feeling a little uncomfortable after the drive." He asked a lot of questions and continued to probe, though I tried to brush it off. As the crushing pain stayed, I broke down and said, "I'm having chest pain." With deeply concerned eyes looking down from his 6'6" frame, Kevin focused deep into my worried eyes. "Dee, describe the pain and tell me how long this has been happening." I told him everything I could remember and felt heard.

Kevin then moved me gently over to the couch to lie down and rest. He kneeled beside the couch on one knee. I thought, "Oh no, is he going to propose now?" Okay, that's not what he did. But I will never forget what happened next, and I'll always hold it close to me. He put his hand lightly on my chest and prayed for me. I never felt more cared about by him than at that moment.

As special as the moment was...the pain in my chest still hung around. Eventually it subsided. I didn't eat and took his delicious meal home. We spent our time mostly in silence. Him worrying and doting on me and me just a little afraid to drive back home.

I had never felt anything remotely similar to the crushing pain that lasted for more than forty-five minutes. Still, it didn't occur to Kevin or me that this, coupled with the swollen feet and ankles, had anything to do with my heart. Not one bell, whistle, or air horn went off in my head. None of it connected for me.

### Denise's Words of Wisdom (WOW)

**Believe in Something Bigger than yourself:** I'm a Christian. I believe in prayer and now know that Kevin does too. We had never discussed it, prior to his kneeling next to me to pray. Survival of anything means you have to believe in something bigger than your current circumstances to get through it.

**Signs of an underlying heart issue.** Different symptoms can indicate different types of heart disease. Be aware of these signs that might seem insignificant but could signal that your heart health is at risk:

### ◆ Extreme fatigue

**Yes,** there are many conditions that can cause fatigue. However, persistent, unexplained tiredness could be a sign that your heart is not pumping well or is encountering some other problem—like a blockage or a valve issue.

### ◆ Shortness of breath

Sure, you get winded easily if you're a little out of shape, but don't be so quick to shrug it off. If you find yourself gasping for air after a small amount of exertion, like walking out to the car or up the front steps, it might be your heart.

### ◆ Digestive concerns

Lightheadedness, nausea, vomiting, or stomach pain can be common signs of a heart attack—especially for women, who often have different symptoms than men. It can start with a vague sense of not feeling well in the digestive area or heartburn, but these, along with breaking into a cold sweat, can indicate something far greater than an upset stomach.

### ◆ Trouble sleeping

This isn't just an every now and then you can't get to sleep or back to sleep. I'm talking about sleep apnea (snoring, waking up during the night). Heart disease could be behind your poor night's sleep. Your blood flow and heart rate change when you go to sleep when everything is functioning normally. If there's something wrong, it could be waking you up at 1 a.m. Heart failure can cause sleep apnea or make fluid build-up in the lungs. Arrhythmia can make you feel like your heart is racing. Heart failure and arrhythmia can interrupt your sleep and be an indication something is wrong with your heart.

- Swelling

This can be a sign of heart failure, especially in the legs, ankles, or feet. If you have puffed up so much that your finger leaves an indent when you touch your body, you should probably check with your medical professional. Sudden swelling is not because you're overweight.

- Chest discomfort or angina

Feelings of squeezing, tightness, pressure, or heaviness can be signals that something is wrong with your heart.

People commonly describe cardiac distress as feeling like an elephant is sitting on their chest.

◆ **Leg cramps**

Leg pain, or difficulty walking, can be a sign that your circulation is impaired. The main organ behind blood flow is your heart.

◆ **Heart rhythm and rate changes**

When your heartbeat feels unusual—too fast or uneven—that is called palpitations. It's a feeling similar to when you've had too much caffeine or feel panicked. But if you're just sitting and reading a book, and your heart starts to race, it could mean you're at risk for heart disease.

◆ **Shoulder, arm, neck, back, abdomen, or jaw pain**

When your heart is on the struggle bus, it can make other parts of your body scream out in pain. Arm pain is a classic heart attack symptom, but it can also occur in the shoulders, back, stomach, or jaw.

◆ **Dizziness or lightheadedness**

Feeling faint usually means there's not enough blood flow to the brain. There can be many causes, and abnormal heart function could be one of them—especially when you feel dizzy upon standing up.

◆ **Persistent cough**

Heart failure can make fluid build-up in your lungs, which can trigger coughing or wheezing.

# CHAPTER THREE

# TIME FOR AN OIL CHANGE

## *Warning Signs of a Heart Attack*

*Having a car is cool until you have to get an oil change, an inspection, a registration sticker, new tires, or pay for gas.*
*—Unknown*

My sentiments exactly. Everything is well and good until you need to have work done. I can remember depending on the little sticker they would put in the upper left corner of the windshield after an oil change. Seriously, without the sticker I usually don't pay attention to the mileage enough to know when I've hit the recommended 3,000 to 5,000 miles to have the oil changed. If for some reason they missed adding the sticker or it fell off, I was lost. It would take smelling oil outside of the car, exhaust smoke, or as a last resort a change engine oil light. Fortunately, my current car lets me know pretty early that I will need an oil change. It even says, "change oil soon."

Have you ever run out of gas because you kept driving while the fuel indicator was close to empty? How about seeing exhaust smoke because you didn't pay attention to the "change oil" light? Just like your car needs regular maintenance to keep it from breaking down, so does your body. Unbeknownst to me, I was getting "maintenance needed" signs but missing them entirely. My body was warning me with swollen feet and ankles, chest pain, and shortness of breath. The next sign would come from an unexpected source...new patient paperwork for my seventy-two-year-old mother!

Mother has always been the picture of health. She tells me that as a child and into her teens, she was super skinny and a little sickly. She was anemic and every now and then would faint. Back then they would use smelling salts or a stinky shoe to bring her back. Never a hospitalization or call to the doctor. But as an adult, outside of a sinus infection, my mom didn't get sick. I couldn't tell you the last time she went to a doctor. Not even a primary care physician for a checkup. Her mantra was "I don't take any meds, and God keeps me well." I'm not pushing the narrative of not seeing a doctor. If you're the picture of health, then let a doctor confirm you're healthy.

After years of my uncle and brother asking Mom to simply get checked out, she relented and found a doctor. What finally pushed her over the wall was a letter from Medicare laying out all the reasons she should and needed to see a physician. It bordered on mandating she go to a doctor.

Mother went through the arduous task of picking a physician in the Humana network. The doctor's office sent over a litany of new patient paperwork. They didn't direct her to go online but instead actually mailed it. As we sat down to tackle it, I was impressed at the level of thoroughness. The information was incredibly organized—every part had a section to complete:

» Ear, nose, throat
» Ophthalmology
» Mental
» Internal
» Osteoporosis

Buried somewhere between how many surgeries she had, and the number of live births was the cardiac section. We were on a roll. She didn't have any check marks next to any of the symptoms. No shortness of breath, no swollen extremities, no chest pain. Gold star for Mom but not for me.

As I read the symptom of swollen feet and ankles, inside I was screaming, "I knew damn well my feet weren't swelling just because I'm fat!" As I sat with Mom, my feet were still swollen. We finished her paperwork with barely any check marks. She was ready for her appointment...and I knew I needed to find a cardiologist.

It was my turn to complete the laborious task of finding a cardiologist in my network. It never occurred to me to ask anyone for a recommendation. I could have asked my primary care physician, but I wasn't talking to Dr. Challa. The "swollen feet because you're fat" comment was still bothersome for me. I didn't know what my criteria should be for finding a cardiologist. I thought I wanted a female and knew I wanted her to care a lot about women's heart health.

There was a myriad of female cardiologists in Frisco, TX. I narrowed my search down to one African-American and two Caucasians. I called the office of the African-American first. She had decent enough reviews. I described my symptoms. The office manager had an incredible amount of urgency in her voice. She said, "We need to get you in as soon as possible to see Dr.

Johnson." It was Thursday, and my appointment was set for the following Tuesday, April 28, 2015. I thought, "This is surely a sign I've found the right one."

Bummer, there was not any new patient paperwork to fill in prior to my appointment. When I arrived what I filled out amounted to signing my name as the person responsible for the bill and to acknowledge all payments were due upon service. I can remember the appointment like it was yesterday.

# Chapter Four

# The Appointment

## Diagnosing Heart Disease

*"A thousand words will not leave
so deep an impression as one deed."*
—Henrik Ibsen

*"A thousand words will not leave
so deep an impression as one deed or the lack of a deed."*
—Denise Castille

The day I met Dr. Johnson I wore a pair of wide leg pants and a sleeveless top. Still reeling from the fat insult from Dr. Challa, I didn't dare bare my floppy arms. I had them covered with a beautiful jacket. My feet were visibly swollen and looked like two pregnant pigs in really cute shoes, but I had to wear those skinny heels into the office. I might have heart issues, but I was hell bent on being cute!

The heart disease, angina, lower your cholesterol, high blood pressure posters littered the walls like they were trying way too hard to make a case. At the front desk I recognized her voice...it was the office manager who said I needed to get in for an appointment as soon as possible. She believed my very life depended on getting in sooner than later...BUT she wasn't the doctor.

I had only been there a short time when Dr. Johnson's nurse came to get me. It wasn't lost on me that those same posters about heart health for women, a condition called angina, taking a baby aspirin, and lowering your cholesterol were down the hallways and in the examination room I was taken to. Before she opened her folder and took one note she asked me a question I thought was strictly reserved for department stores, "What brings you in today?" There were no assumptions that just because I had told the office manager about my swollen feet and ankles, shortness of breath, and chest pain that I was in a cardiologist's office for heart related issues. I described my symptoms in detail. I went all the way back to my swollen feet. I included all of the remedies I had tried and about the chest pain. The nurse asked routine information like did I smoke, about pregnancies, and my drinking habits.

Soon, Dr. Johnson walked in. Her name was prominently displayed on her white lab coat, but this did not look at all like the person on the Internet. Clearly, she was using a very dated picture as her profile. Between the look of the office and her aging appearance I joked to myself, "How out of date is her medical practice? Will she use leeches to treat my swollen feet?!!"

She introduced herself and limply shook my hand. We didn't have a lot of banter. She re-asked a lot of the same questions as her nurse. She looked at my ankles and commented, "You should wear more sensible shoes" as though my skinny heels had caused the swelling. She told me, "You need to be on a low sodium diet to get rid of the swelling. I suggest 2,000 mg of sodium per day." There was no dialogue about any connection swollen feet might have to a heart condition.

Dr. Johnson rattled off her comments without so much as a glimmer of personality. She wasn't the least bit pleasant. I thought, "Maybe she just needs to warm up to me." I barely heard her when she said, "The nurse will be back to do an EKG." Honestly, I was still at "You should wear more sensible shoes" and the lack of pleasantries. Her bedside manner sucked.

The nurse was back asking me to lift up my shirt and spanx so she could attach twelve small plastic patches to my chest,

29

abdomen, and upper arm area. Great, now they're going to know I don't have a tiny waist. "Hold on a minute! What, are we doing?" I asked. The nurse said, "Dr. Johnson wants to do an EKG." It was quick. She told me to lie still, and I held my breath. The nurse printed out the activity of my heart for my doctor to measure and interpret.

She had my results. They were abnormal. Shame on her for not telling me what might cause an abnormal EKG. And, of course, shame on me for not asking what might make it abnormal. She never said during a heart attack, blood flow in the heart is affected and heart tissue can begin to lose oxygen and die. This tissue will not conduct electricity as well, which can cause an abnormal EKG. Ischemia or lack of blood flow may also cause an abnormal EKG.[3] (found in Healthline.com). The nurse explained Dr. Johnson wanted me to have a stress test that they could conduct right there in the office. I asked her, "Am I having a stress test because of the abnormal EKG?" She responded, "No, you're having a stress test because of the chest pain you complained about." She ushered me down the hall to the "stress technician."

-------------------

[3] *"Heart Attack." Retrieved from*
*https://www.healthline.com/health/heart-attack#symptoms*

## The Stress Test

The stress test technician was by far the most verbose and thorough of the staff. She said, "The test is used to determine what your heart does when it is subjected to physical activity. A *stress* test makes your heart work harder." I thought they should call the test what it is—an *exercise* test. The test is administered on a treadmill or stationary bicycle. Mine was on a treadmill. The technician said, "Your blood pressure could drop dangerously low causing you to faint, your heart could beat irregularly (called an arrhythmia), or though rare, you could suffer a heart attack or even die." She reiterated I would need to wear loose fitting clothes and fast prior to the appointment. "Won't fasting make me more susceptible to passing out?" Her response came quickly. "We'll be here if something happens." Didn't quite answer my question.

I came in for the hour-long stress test. I know why they call it a stress test—it stresses the hell out of you! Some heart problems are easier to identify when your heart is working hard to pump blood throughout your body, such as when you exercise. A stress test is recommended when there are symptoms of a heart problem such as shortness of breath, chest pain, dizziness, and a rapid or irregular heartbeat.[4] I certainly had symptoms.

The technician had been very thorough explaining what to expect. As the test progressed, they wanted me to stay on the treadmill a lot longer as they increased the speed and the incline. I couldn't, which just said to me...I am out of shape. Finally, it was over, and I was drinking apple juice and having a few of those orange crackers with peanut butter between them.

### Hail Damage

I can spot hail damage on a car a mile away. I worked for State Farm insurance for ten years. I was on the Auto Catastrophe team, also handled roof damage, and inspected thousands of cars and hundreds of roofs. There were times when my inspections came up with zero damage. Good news, right? Rarely were insureds happy about not having damage. Delivering the news was hardest with men. They would demand that I come back to their car while they pointed out an

--------------------

[4] *"EKGs and Stress Tests: When You Need Them—and When You Don't." (2012, April). Retrieved from* https://www.choosingwisely.org/patient-resources/ekgs-and-exercise-stress-tests/

imperfection, but it was not hail damage. Others would show me minor damage that in actuality was nothing to speak of.

On May 15th, one week after the stress test, I was back in the office for the results. I expected to hear there was "hail damage" or what "body repair" needed to be done. Dr. Johnson walked in with the same overall dull look on her face. She said, "Great news, you don't have any blockage or valve problems." How on earth do you deliver great news without so much as a smile? I did not feel convinced there was no damage.

My stress test was done to give the doctor important information about the likelihood of a heart problem. She had just told me there was 0% likelihood I was headed for or had heart issues. This is good, right? I said, "Just so I'm clear, the stress test is designed to find out if I have blockage or valves problems?" She replied, "Yes, it determines if one or more of the coronary arteries is more than 70% blocked." "And I have 0% blockage?" "Yes, there is no blockage or valves problems," she repeated.

| Test Result[5] | What it Could Mean | What Could Still Happen | Next Steps |
|---|---|---|---|
| Normal | You do not have significant coronary artery disease (70% or greater blockage) | You could still have a heart attack if a smaller blockage (70% ruptures and forms a clot) | Your doctor may want to do further testing if you have other risk factors for heart disease that are raising concern |
| Abnormal | You may have significant coronary artery disease (70% or greater blockage) | The abnormal result may be a false alarm and could require further testing to confirm | Your doctor may order additional tests to confirm that you have coronary artery disease |

I wanted to feel relieved. I didn't want to be the unhappy insured with my non-hail damage estimate...but hell, this was my heart. "What about my abnormal EKG? Did it matter

---

[5] *"Cardiac Exercise Stress Testing: What It Can and Cannot Tell You."* *(2020, April 15). Retrieved from* *https://www.health.harvard.edu/heart-disease-overview/cardiac-exercise-stress-testing-what-it-can-and-cannot-tell-you*

anymore? Was it a false positive? The chest pain was a fluke? There isn't anything else to do? No more tests?" It would have been great for me to stop asking myself these questions in my head and ask Dr. Johnson. She bid me farewell before I had the courage to ask the questions out loud. At this point I made a serious mistake. I didn't look for another doctor, despite the fact we didn't get along at all, I didn't respect her, and I didn't trust her opinions on my test results. My decision would have serious consequences.

### Denise's Words of Wisdom (WOW)

**There are other tests.** I thought Dr. Johnson had administered the one and only test available to determine if there was blockage. Here are the tests [6]your cardiologist can conduct and why:

1. **Echocardiogram:** Uses sound waves to produce images of your heart. This common test allows your physician to see how your heart is beating and how blood is moving through your heart. Images from an echocardiogram are

---

[6] *"10 Heart Tests Your Doctor Might Order, and What They Mean."* *(2020, February 3). Retrieved from* *https://healthblog.uofmhealth.org/heart-health/10-heart-tests-your-doctor-might-order-and-what-they-mean*

used to identify various abnormalities in the heart muscle and valves. This test can be done while you're at rest or with exercise to elevate your heart rate.

**Reasons for the test:**

>> Determine the cause of a heart murmur

>> Check the function of heart valves

>> Assess the overall function of the heart

2. **Transesophageal echocardiography (TEE):** Uses high-frequency sound waves (ultrasound) to make detailed pictures of your heart and the arteries that lead to and from it. The echo transducer that produces the sound waves for TEE is attached to a thin tube that passes through your mouth, down your throat, and into your esophagus, which is very close to the upper chambers of the heart.

**Reasons for the test:**

>> Assess the function of heart valves

>> Follow heart valve disease

>> Look for blood clots inside the heart

3. **Electrocardiogram (ECG or EKG):** Measures the electrical activity of the heartbeat to provide two kinds of information. First, by measuring time intervals of the ECG, a doctor can determine how long the electrical wave takes to pass through your heart. Finding out how

long a wave takes to travel from one part of the heart to the next shows if the electrical activity is normal, slow, fast, or irregular. Second, by measuring the amount of electrical activity passing through your heart muscle, a cardiologist may be able to find out if parts of the heart are too large or overworked.

**Reasons for the test:**

>> Monitor changes in heart rhythm
>> Determine whether a heart attack has occurred
>> Help predict if a heart attack is developing

4. **Magnetic resonance imaging (MRI):** Uses a magnetic field and radiofrequency waves to create detailed pictures of organs and structures inside your body. It can be used to examine your heart and blood vessels and to identify areas of the brain affected by stroke.

**Reasons for the test:**

>> Assess heart structure
>> Look for scar tissue within the heart muscle
>> Assess the function of heart valves

5. **Ct scan:** An x-ray imaging technique that uses a computer to produce cross-sectional images of your heart. Also referred to as cardiac computed tomography, computerized axial tomography, or CAT scan, it can be used to examine your heart and blood vessels for

problems. It's also used to identify whether blood vessels in the brain have been affected by stroke.

**Reasons for the test:**

>> Assess the structure of the heart

>> Determine if blockages are present in the coronary arteries

6. **Exercise cardiac stress test:** Also called an exercise tolerance test (ETT), this test shows whether your heart's blood supply is sufficient and if your heart rhythm is normal during exercise on a treadmill or stationary bicycle. The test monitors your level of tiredness, heart rate, breathing, blood pressure, and heart activity while exercising. This test may be done in combination with nuclear imaging or echocardiography.

**Reasons for the test:**

>> Determine the cause of chest pain, shortness of breath, and weakness

>> Assess the health of the heart

>> Assess safety of exercise

>> Identify heart rhythm changes with activity

>> Find evidence of inadequate blood flow to the heart muscle during exercise

7. **Pharmacologic stress test:** Medication is given through an IV line in your arm to dilate the arteries, which

increases your heart rate and blood flow, similar to the effects of exercise. This test may be done in combination with nuclear imaging, echocardiography, or MRI.

**Reasons for the test:**

>> Determine the cause of chest pain, shortness of breath, and weakness
>> Find evidence of inadequate blood flow to the heart muscle during exercise
>> Monitor or diagnose blockages in the coronary arteries
>> Assess risks for heart attack

8. **Tilt Test:** Often used to determine why you feel faint or lightheaded. During the test, you lie on a table that is slowly tilted upward. The test measures how your blood pressure and heart rate respond to the force of gravity. A nurse or technician keeps track of blood pressure and heart rate (pulse) to see how they change during the test.

**Reasons for the test:**

>> Assess dizziness or fainting spells
>> Identify heart rhythm change

9. **Ambulatory rhythm monitoring tests:** Holter monitoring, event recorders, and mobile cardiac telemetry (MCT) are ambulatory monitoring tests done to study your heart

rhythm for a prolonged period of time. Done on an outpatient basis.

**Reasons for the tests:**
> » Look for evidence of heart rhythm problems that come and go and that are not apparent with a standard ECG

10. **Coronary angiogram:** A type of X-ray used to examine the coronary arteries supplying blood to your heart. A catheter is inserted into a blood vessel in your arm or groin and fed up to your coronary arteries. Special dye is then injected through the catheter and images are taken.

**Results for the tests:**
> » Identify narrowing or blockages in the coronary arteries
> » Evaluate pressures inside the heart

**When your doctor doesn't like you.** It was obvious after a couple of visits that Dr. Johnson and I did not get along. Staying with a doctor who doesn't jive with you can be detrimental. It's okay to change and find one you feel comfortable with, trust, and gives you the care you deserve.

Doctors, of course, are human. They like some people more than others, so it is not surprising that some of my doctors liked me more than others. According to Dr. Jerome Groopman, M.D., in *How Doctors Think*, what's important is that whether a doctor likes or dislikes you can affect your care. He says, "Doctors who like you are more apt to listen to your complaints and take them seriously, rather than jump to conclusions based on generalities that may or may not apply. Worse, by not listening to you may mean a doctor could miss or misdiagnose important symptoms."[7]

---

[7] *Groopman, M.D. Jerome (2007). How Doctors Think. Houghton Mifflin.*

# Chapter Five

# A Mile High
# and Misdiagnosed

## Heart Attack Misdiagnosis and Delayed Diagnosis

*"Usually doctors are right, but conservatively about 15% of all people are misdiagnosed. Some experts think it's as high as 20% to 25%."*
—Jerome Groopman, M.D.

During this time of doctor visits and testing, I was traveling close to 85% for work. I know that work travel can be stressful, but for the most part mine was uneventful. This trip was going to be laid back in comparison to other trips. I didn't have to rent a car or drive. I rode with Clarke, from the office, while we were in the mile-high city of Denver,

Colorado. Almost as soon as we arrived, I started having symptoms of shortness of breath and a new one—palpitations.

I had started taking my blood pressure twice a day just after my last appointment on May 15th. My sixth sense told me to keep track of how I was feeling, my blood pressure, what I did, what I ate, my activities—everything. I was still experiencing shortness of breath along with swollen feet.

Half way through the week I called Dr. Johnson's office. I spoke with the nurse. Before she scheduled the follow-up, she must have looked up my chart because she commented that my stress test didn't show any heart issues. She took the time to say, "Sometimes people are so in tune with their bodies that they misinterpret regular heart beats as palpitations. It's normal for the heartbeat to get up to 100 beats per minute. The palpitations could be from drinking too much caffeine, you might be having a panic attack, or just plain ole stressed." I learned a lot about palpitations in the short conversation with the nurse. After I spoke with her, I took every measure to not stress or elevate my heart rate.

My appointment was scheduled for June 12th, and a little over a week had passed since I made the appointment. The palpitations weren't stopping, and I kept track of everything on a spreadsheet. They were so intense, for the first time ever I thought about my heart all the time.

When I arrived for my appointment, I had three copies of the spreadsheet—one for Dr. Johnson, the nurse, and me. I gave the nurse two copies of the spreadsheet. "One for you and one for Dr. Johnson," I said. The nurse seemed impressed. In about ten minutes, Dr. Johnson came in without even a greeting. She was clearly frustrated. It felt like I was intruding on her time, though I had made an appointment. I expected that Dr. Johnson and I would review my spreadsheet, but instead she started to hand it back to me. I quickly said, "That one is yours. I have one." She responded, "I don't need this because there is nothing wrong with your heart." I was completely taken aback by her declaration that there was nothing wrong with me. I felt frustrated after the work I had done. I had this overwhelming sense of rejection. There were no follow up questions regarding my spreadsheet. I mentioned palpitations. She didn't ask what the heart palpitations felt like or if I was still experiencing shortness of breath after my return from Denver. How was it possible there was nothing wrong with me? I felt like crap.

This appointment I was assertive and asked, "Could you explain why I am experiencing palpitations? She breathed hard and said, "You're just stressed." The look on my face surely must have screamed something because she said with an uncompromising tone and a little louder, "There is nothing wrong with your heart." Now, she was just being rude. Again, she emphasized, "You might be a little stressed, but that's it."

As my eyes roamed the walls reading about taking an aspirin and heart disease, I wanted to scream, "Should I take an aspirin, just in case? What about angina—do I have that?" I still wasn't armed with a lot of information about heart disease or heart attack symptoms to be a strong advocate for myself. I didn't need the Internet to know I wasn't feeling well. It certainly didn't help that Dr. Johnson and I didn't have a good doctor/patient relationship. There I was back in her office with some serious complaints. Consistent high blood pressure, shortness of breath, and palpitations. She was bothered by me and didn't offer to take the next step with another test. I had paid my $50 co-pay for a specialty office visit with a doctor I should have left weeks ago.

About 1.5 million heart attacks occur in the United States each year, and studies show that about 11,000 cases are not properly diagnosed, resulting in unnecessary deaths.[8]  It is imperative that you ask questions regarding your heart health.

### Denise's Words of Wisdom (WOW)

**Prepare for your visit with the doctor.** Contrary to Dr. Johnson's actions, you should absolutely prepare for your visit with the cardiologist (or any doctor).

» Compile a personal health history and a health history of your family.

» Gather together any **recent test results** and a **list of medications** you are taking.

» Jot down notes about **symptoms** you have been experiencing.

» Make a **list of questions** you want to ask your doctor.

**Explain your symptoms.** I am like most people. I do not like visits to the doctor (outside the big five at the start of the year). If I make an appointment outside of the regularly scheduled annual ones—it's serious. Don't allow the doctor to generalize

[8] *"Heart Attack Misdiagnosis and Delayed Diagnosis." Retrieved from https://www.seattlemalpracticelawyers.com/legal-services/medical-malpractice-lawyer/heart-attack-delayed-misdiagnosis/*

your symptoms. She or he has never treated these symptoms in YOUR body.

**Make sure your questions are answered.** This is very important, even if you feel nervous to ask or aren't familiar with medical issues. Most people are just like you. Make sure your questions are answered and in a way that you understand. It's okay to say, "Could you please explain that in more simple terms? I'm interested in what you have to say and learning more." Most doctors won't object to patients who want to learn how to take better care of themselves.

# Chapter Six

# The Delay

## Minutes Matter in Getting Treatment for a Heart Attack

*"Sometimes you are delayed where you are because God knows there's a storm where you're headed. Be grateful!"*
*—Unknown*

"Women are more likely than men to die from a heart attack due to delays in treatment," according to a study presented at the American College of Cardiology's 64th Annual Scientific Session in San Diego, CA. "Delays in treatment have a major impact on survival rates for women. Women suffering a heart attack were nearly twice as likely to die in the hospital compared to men, with in-hospital deaths reported for twelve percent of women and six percent of men in the study. Women were also less likely to undergo treatment to open clogged arteries, which can be lifesaving when performed soon after the heart attack starts.[9]"

My next work trip was planned for the week of June 29th. I was headed to the thriving metropolis of Detroit. My job as a Corporate Operations Advisor for a janitorial franchisor often meant a lot of clean up (no pun intended) work. I arrived in Detroit and hit the ground running. There were big clients to appease with a myriad of promises to have their offices and restaurants cleaned to as close to perfection as possible.

A long-time friend Maurice and I met for dinner and to catch up. We went to one of my favorites—Outback Steak House. No aussie chips or blooming onion for me, though. I ordered the salmon with broccoli. After talking for a while, I shared my current situation—chest pain, heart palpitations, and swollen feet. His face was grim as I laid out the symptoms. I told him, "The doctor assured me that it is just stress, and there is nothing wrong with my heart." It looked like he wasn't buying it in the

---
[9] *"Delays in Treatment Worsen Heart Attack Outcomes in Women." (2015, March 16). Retrieved from* https://www.cardiosmart.org/news/2015/3/delays-in-treatment-worsen-heart-attack-outcomes-in-women

least bit. Maurice said, "If you say so. Do you think you should get a second opinion?" In addition to my mistake of not changing doctors sooner, I also didn't seek another doctor's opinion when I knew there was something wrong and my pain continued. Two very hard lessons to learn that thankfully have become opportunities to help others and myself in our journey to better health.

I woke up in Farmington Hills, MI, a suburb of Detroit, on Thursday, July 2, 2015. It was early, had a super busy day ahead, and I was excited to get back to Dallas. I had a date, it was the 4th of July holiday weekend, and the long week had worn me out.

I grabbed a quick bite for breakfast and was in the car headed to my first appointment by about 6:15 a.m. I know I did more than six inspections before lunch. I was in route to a couple of poorly cleaned car dealerships when I received a call from Tanya, the Assistant Director of the department. "Call me when you get to the airport." I pleaded with her, "This must be important. Please tell me now." She said briefly, "I'm leaving the company." I ended the call with, "I promise to call you back once I got to the airport." I couldn't believe Tanya was leaving. She was the lifeblood of the department. We hadn't known each other long, but we had become good friends. It made me sad to think about her leaving.

The next several appointments went off without a hitch. The last appointment included Carlos, the Detroit Regional Director. We made a lot of promises in the meeting, came out, and parted ways. Carlos had a stop to make before heading to the office. I was starving and decided to stop as soon as something grabbed me. Arby's was calling me. I got my food and pulled into a parking space to chat with my mom and also ensure she would be at the airport on time.

As I continued to talk with my mom, it happened... The biggest heart palpitation I had ever felt came and lingered. I gasped with surprise, and it took my breath away. Mom commented without my telling her what had happened. She said, "Niecy, you've got to get that checked out." I retorted, "Ma, I already did...the doctor said it's just stress." I confirmed Mom would be at the airport and said, "I love you." She said, "God be with you," her special way of saying she loves me.

I drove back to work with a renewed since of urgency. I had taken too long eating and chatting with Mom. I would have to hurry to get everything done and to the airport on time. I pulled into the office complex, the parking lot nearly empty from people leaving early for the holiday weekend.

As I walked to my office, I got a text message that my flight was delayed by a little more than an hour. I felt deflated to have to wait, but what can you do? I sighed and was glad to see I wasn't alone. Carlos had beaten me back and stopped to chat. He was dressed in his baseball regalia and said, "I'm headed to pick up my kids and off to a game." We talked briefly about my schedule and plans to return the following week. He said, "I don't want you to worry with an Uber or taxi, so take the company car you're driving and leave it at the airport parking lot." "Thanks, Carlos. I won't have to take my luggage out and can just drive myself." Last thing he said as he walked out... "Marsha is still here and the only one in the office. I'll see you Monday afternoon." As he closed the door I yelled, "Have a good holiday!" He heard me and yelled back, "You too, and have a good flight!"

I had accomplished so much during the week, and now I had time to complete my reports and return some calls. I had checked everything off my list and thought, "Perfect timing." Now, I would head to the airport.

As I was gathering my things and clearing off the desk, I heard the bothersome chirp that I had a text message. I just knew it was the airline noting another delay. I turned to reach for the phone but never saw the text. I gasped not from a palpitation but something that was far worse. I felt as though I was suffocating, and I couldn't catch my breath. I didn't know what it was, but I needed to shake it off and get to the airport.

It was far worse than when I was on my way to Kevin's house. I stood up, but the weight of whatever it was pushed me back into my seat. By now I was sweating profusely and felt I was about to pass out. In retrospect, I was still doing it—ignoring obvious signs that something was wrong. I shudder to think what could have happened if I had somehow managed to shake it off and head to the airport.

I mustered up the strength to stand again and keep standing. I struggled to make it to the door and out to the common office space. I cried out, "Marsha?" She responded, "Are you headed to the airport?" All I could say was, "No, I don't feel well." Marsha ran out, saw me, and ran back shouting, "I'm calling 911."

When Marsha got back to me, I was on the floor. I felt delirious and losing touch with what was happening around me. She was on the phone with the 911 dispatch. As they asked her questions, she talked to me. She said, "The paramedics are on their way." I whispered, "They better hurry." With the phone still to her ear, she said, "Denise, I have to let the paramedics in. Keep breathing, stay with me."

While Marsha was gone I prayed, *"God please don't let me die like this...I don't want to die like this."* There were times I was unaware of my own existence or surroundings. My awareness of time was going in and out. I don't remember the paramedics putting the EKG leads on me, but I do remember hearing one of them shout, "We gotta go. She's positive for MI." I didn't know what MI was, but I knew whatever it was caused intense pain. I wanted them to make the MI stop. I would later learn that MI meant myocardial infarction (heart attack).

The paramedics were running with the gurney. They loaded me into the ambulance. I heard sirens blaring and a driver honking his horn in long nonstop succession. We arrived at the hospital to a scene that mirrored a *Grey's Anatomy* episode. The emergency room team had been alerted that a patient was actively having an MI, and the ambulance was en route. The paramedics came in and said what they encountered. Just before they left, one of them grabbed my shoeless foot and said, "Good luck Ms. Castille."

I began to lose track of time—but it felt like a short time later the ER doctor came over, leaned in close to me and said, "You're having a heart attack, and we're going to do everything we can to help you." The medical staff seemed to work at lightning speed. They took a pair of scissors and cut my clothes off. Someone grabbed my phone and dialed the last number. It was my mom. The doctor apprised her of the situation. Months later Mom shared her reaction as feeling paralyzed with fear and confusion. She tried to make sense of it—how would she get to me when I was so far away? By the time my brother called her back, she was crying uncontrollably. He said, "Ma, we have to pray." She prayed for healing and direction.

Someone asked me if I had taken any drugs. "No, I haven't, not ever." Wait, I thought I was having a heart attack. Now, do they think I've overdosed on drugs? I had an oxygen mask on and wasn't even sure I was answering their questions. I now know the question about drugs had to be asked. According to research by the American Heart Association (AHA), cocaine is the illegal drug most associated with visits to emergency departments. Cocaine use has been associated with chest pain and myocardial infarction.[10] Someone else was looking through my purse for what, I'm not sure. The whole time I didn't care that I was naked or that they were going through my belongings. This medical team was moving at high speed, and I just wanted them to quickly get the freakin' elephant off my chest or even raise him up a tad.

Have you, or someone you care for, ever experienced a heart attack or something similar? The feeling of something heavy on your chest is indescribable—the best I can do is say it

---

[10] *"Illegal Drugs and Heart Disease." Retrieved from https://www.heart.org/en/health-topics/consumer-healthcare/what-is-cardiovascular-disease/illegal-drugs-and-heart-diseaselooking*

is akin to suffocating. I felt outside my body thinking, "There are people all around. Why can't they move whatever is on my chest off of it?" There were moments of darkness where I felt as though I was falling into an abyss. Was I going to die?

A nurse was doing a good job of talking to me and telling me what was happening. They were running and pushing my bed at the same time. I soon was in a super cold room. They must have given me something because I felt really subdued. The pain was still catastrophic; I was mentally drifting but conscious enough to be somewhat aware of activity around me. The doctor made an incision in my groin and inserted something. I found out later he had opened the blocked artery to my heart and inserted two coated stents to keep the artery open. A short while later the elephant was lifted—slightly and then completely. When the weight was completely lifted off my chest the doctor said, "You feel better don't you?" I smiled and nodded yes.

Another nurse remarked, "Let's get you to your room—I'm sure you've got family waiting for you." Suddenly I realized, "I'm alone in this city. There's no family to come one by one to ICU." I told her, "I live in Dallas and was only here for work." She was very surprised by my statement and replied, "We'll be your family." I'm not sure what it was about that moment versus the tremendous pain I endured or thinking I was going to die—but I cried for the first time. I was lying flat on my back, and the tears dropped from the corners of my eyes.

They rolled my bed to ICU. The male nurse eagerly introduced himself and told me, "I will take good care of you." It started with the ER doctor telling me they would do everything they could to help me, the nurse who said they would be my family, and now this nurse vowing to take good care of me. They were great at keeping their promises. He shared that my sister was on her way from Fort Wayne, IN. I had no idea who he was talking about. He said, "I talked to your mom, and she assured me your sister is on her way." Maybe the morphine and any of the other medical cocktails they had given me was confusing me, but I was sure I heard him say my sister. I don't have a sister...

Not sure where the miscommunication was, but my cousin Terrie arrived. She was a nurse and lived in Fort Wayne. My cousin had driven to be by my side despite not having a charged phone, making navigation even more problematic, and battled road construction. She was prepared to stay until the next day when she would leave for work.

Naturally, Terrie started asking medical questions like, "How much morphine has Denise been given?" I was in and out of consciousness, but I remember the male nurse nicely ask Terrie,

"Are you in the medical profession?" She proudly said, "Yes." Thankfully, he said in the kindest possible way, "We've got it. You can just hold her hand." Terrie reluctantly stopped asking questions and did hold my hand.

At some point during the night, two doctors came in to tell me that I was about to go through a tremendous amount of pain with the procedure of taking the sheath out that had been put in my groin to hold the stents. The narrative was delivered with deliberate poignancy, expressing regret for the pain I would feel. They told me, "You will need to lie flat for about six hours. Then we will come in and apply manual pressure to the wound to remove the sheath." I appreciated how forthcoming they were with the description. I felt as though I could brace myself for what they were going to do.

Terrie was also descriptive and held nothing back. In my childlike voice I asked, "Will you stay with me?" She asked the nurse and two doctors if she could stay. They unequivocally told her, "No."

The doctors had told the truth...it hurt. However, the pain was minor in comparison with the earlier elephant that sat on my chest. I thought, "I'm learning a lot through this crappy and painful experience. Nobody should go through what I have."

I looked up and through the door was another Terri. It was my bestie and her husband Paul! "What are you both doing here? How did you know?" Paul made me chuckle with their answer. He said, "Terri got the call while watching an episode of *Law & Order: Special Victims Unit.* She hung up from your mom and told me 'We are driving to Detroit tonight!' In record time Terri's bag was packed, and she was at the door. I reasoned with her that since it was after 10 p.m., maybe we should wait until daybreak. She rolled her eyes, gave me a big sigh 'Okay, Paul,' and at the crack of dawn she drove like crazy to be here with you."

Dr. Roger and his team came in. Terri asked, "How much blockage did my best friend have? Dr. Roger replied, "There was 99% blockage, and she had the *widow-maker.*" Terri was well versed in hearts and blockage because her mom has been plagued with heart issues. I hadn't spent time studying heart disease, so terms like blockage, stents, and widow-maker were new to me. I remember Dr. Johnson proclaiming I didn't have any blockage or valve problems, so I didn't understand how it got to 99% in less than a month. I was still relatively high on morphine, so I just let everything sink in.

Heart attacks can be fatal, and the widow-maker is the deadliest kind. It can happen suddenly when an artery is blocked preventing blood from getting to the heart. Even though the name suggests the widow-maker only happens in men, it also occurs in women. Your heart muscle needs a constant supply of blood. When the flow is cut off, a heart attack takes place. Without the needed oxygen, the cells in the heart muscles begin to die. Specifically, a widow-maker is a big blockage at the beginning of the left main artery or the left anterior descending artery (LAD). This is the major pipeline for blood. If the blood flow gets 100% blocked at this critical location, it could turn fatal without emergency care. If not for the quick response of Marsha, the paramedics, and the ER team, I may not have survived.

I don't remember the order that the visitors came in but Carlos, the Regional Director, stopped by. He told me, "Tanya is a wreck. She called me and thought you were at the airport about to board your flight." That made sense because she had no idea my flight had been delayed. I found out later she called my mom and left a message, but because Mom doesn't listen to her voicemail, the message remains to this day unheard.

I told Carlos I would be back to the office as soon as they released me from the hospital. He said, "I don't think you'll be coming back quite so soon." He didn't argue with me. He probably knew I was highly medicated. Carlos was right on both counts. I didn't realize my recovery would not only be physical but mental as well. As much as I wanted to bounce back, I had to take time for some self-care that would end up benefitting every part of my life.

It was the next day that Dr. Roger came to my room with a fellow cardiologist and a couple of medical students. They asked me question after question. "Have you ever smoked?" "No." "Used drugs?" I wanted to say, "If I don't get out of here soon, I may start!" I replied, "No. Never." Their questions were coming in rapid succession. I stopped them in their tracks simply by saying, "I visited a cardiologist on June 12th and confirmed I didn't have any blockage or valve problems." Dr. Roger demanded clarification. "Do you mean less than a month ago, June 12th? Or last year, June 12th?" "Doctor, it was a few a weeks ago." He glared and said, "Who in my city has done this?" I gave Dr. Johnson's name. Dr. Roger looked at the other cardiologist and the medical students. The name didn't register with either of them. "I don't live here. This doctor is in Frisco, TX where I live."

They looked more confused. I explained, "I was in town working and was expected on a flight when I developed gut wrenching chest pains." They began to understand, a little. They seemed to still be baffled about the June 12th appointment. "How did the doctor determine there was no blockage or valve problems?" I told them, "She did a stress test and before that an

EKG." They were dumbfounded. Dr. Roger then ordered test after test.

Finally, my mom arrived. She flew to Indianapolis where my uncle and his wife drove her to Detroit. I had survived the widow-maker and was released after several days in ICU. Bestie and Paul had some clothes for me and dropped Mom and I off at the hotel. This would be the first time I stood up on my own. I was glad to have my mom with me in case I needed help. It felt good not to be alone. If washing up was any indication of what my physical recovery was going to be like—I had an uphill battle. It took all of my strength just to take a sink bath. I wouldn't be heading to the office anytime soon...

### Denise's Words of Wisdom (WOW)

**Every minute matters.** Five years to the date after the heart attack, I had an opportunity to speak with the three paramedics who got me to the ER on July 2, 2015. I woke up two days before my five-year *heart-aversary* and said out loud, "I never told them thank you!" I called the fire house that responded to the 911 call and found out the three guys still worked together there. Mom, me, and my three heroes met and talked via Zoom. They said I was their first Zoom "Thank you" meeting. I'm grateful we reunited.

One of the paramedics remembered the call that day. The description was a "weak" person, and he was upset once they arrived because it was far more than "weak." They had to hurry because I was in a full-on heart attack, and time was of the essence. I learned that every minute after a heart attack, more heart tissue deteriorates or dies. Restoring blood flow quickly helps prevent heart damage.

**Go by ambulance.** I didn't have a choice on how I would get to the hospital. Marsha saw my critical situation and wisely decided I was going to the ER by ambulance. I am ashamed to say that there have been times since July 2, 2015 that I have had arguments with Mom over not calling 911. She heard me gasp on the phone, but I brushed her concerned remark off with, "The doctor said it's just stress." I definitely learned the hard way about heart disease and heart attacks and now have many opportunities to educate others how to avoid my mistakes.

I have countless stories about my "heart sisters" who avoided an ambulance and suffered the consequences. Unbeknownst to heart sister, Carrie, she suffered a mini-stroke outside of the United States. She couldn't talk but was shaking her head "No" when asked if she wanted an ambulance. Another gal insisted her husband drive her to ER and tell them she was having a heart attack so she could be seen faster. She didn't know she was actually having one.

Why do we take such chances with our lives? Because we don't want the expensive ambulance bill? We don't want to needlessly bother the paramedics? We are not looking our best? In 2011 a co-worker died in the back of an ambulance from a heart attack. She was in the ambulance but only after her family had pleaded with her. Because every minute matters, it was too late...sadly, time had been wasted persuading her.

**Someone with you.** Even though my cousin Terrie, a nurse, was asking several questions and irritating a few people, she cared about me. You need someone by your side to speak for you when you can't, or you don't know the questions to ask. Find someone to be your voice.

**Heart Attacks.** Acute coronary syndrome (ACS) is when the arteries that carry blood, oxygen, and nutrients get blocked. Heart attacks are a form of ACS. Heart attack is also known as a myocardial infarction (MI). The three types of heart attacks are:

» ST segment elevation myocardial infarction (STEMI)
» Non-ST segment elevation myocardial infarction (NSTEMI)
» Coronary spasm, or unstable angina

**STEMI**: The Classic or Major Heart Attack

People may not know the medical terminology but when you think about a heart attack, it is the STEMI. This heart attack has the classic symptom of pain in the center of the chest. There may be pain in one or both arms, or the back, and jaw.

**NSTEMI** Heart Attack is a partially blocked coronary artery. A NSTEMI won't show any change in the ST segment on the electrocardiogram. A coronary angiography will show the degree to which the artery is blocked. A blood test will also show elevated troponin protein levels. Even though there may be less heart damage, an NSTEMI is still a serious condition.

**Coronary Artery Syndrome** (CAS), silent heart attack or heart attack without blockage, occurs when one of the heart's arteries tightens so much that blood flow stops or becomes drastically reduced. Only imaging and blood test results can tell your doctor if someone has had a silent heart attack. There is no permanent damage during a coronary artery spasm. Even though silent heart attacks are not as serious, they increase the risk of another heart attack or one that is more serious. [11]

------------------------

[11] *"Types of Heart Attacks: What You Should Know." Retrieved from https://www.healthline.com/health/heart-disease/types-of-heart-attacks*

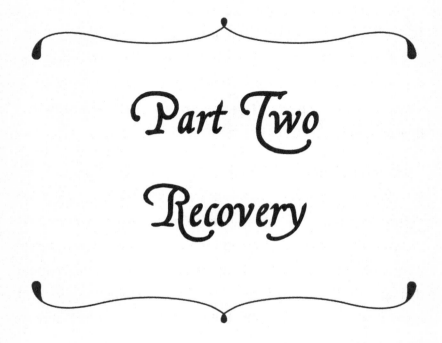

# Part Two

# Recovery

# CHAPTER SEVEN

# READY, SET, GOALS

## Setting Recovery Goals After a Heart Attack

*"Setting goals is the first step*
*in turning the invisible into the visible."*
*—Tony Robbins*

Goal setting is the best way to help with your recovery after a heart attack. Recovery goals help you make important lifestyle changes that can ensure your future health and wellbeing. Goal setting is the best way to keep track of milestones.

> » Set specific goals and write them down
> » Set a plan in motion of how you'll achieve the goal
> » Get support to help you achieve the goal

While I was still in Michigan, Dr. Roger had me take a stress test only days after the heart attack. He described the results as equivalent to "You sitting on a couch flipping through a magazine." My goal was to recover fully to return to work and have more energy and strength than just sitting and flipping through a magazine.

Inactivity increases your risk of developing heart disease. After a heart attack, not moving around isn't good for your heart, either. No matter how you're feeling, it's important to commit to do something every day towards your heart health recovery. Get out of bed and if you feel up to it, make your bed.

Challenge yourself with small, achievable goals and responsibilities. It's important for your goals to matter. Losing weight to prevent heart disease is necessary, but it alone may not be enough motivation. Think about it—you're always tired. No energy and climbing a flight of stairs makes you winded long after you've traversed the stairs. Having more energy may be the motivation you need.

After the heart attack I wanted to eat right, lose weight, exercise more, and volunteer in a way that was impactful. Start off slowly. Pick one and come up with solutions and a plan for achieving the goal. When you pick a goal to achieve, various solutions, and have an action plan, you're much more likely to conquer the goal.

Your recovery goals have to be sensible. It's great to reach for the stars...goals that challenge you. Be mindful of setting goals that are too lofty—trying to reach them might cause you stress. Post heart attack, the goal is to eliminate and diminish stress. Goals that are realistic help to boost your confidence.

When a doctor wants us to lose weight—they usually aren't very specific. They simply tell us to lose weight. If it were that easy, we would have already done it. Ensure your recovery goals are specific.

Give yourself a realistic timetable to complete. It's hard to get and stay motivated when goals are open-ended. Timeframes help move you into action.

Ask for help. Having your healthcare team support boosts your chances for success. According to Healthline, a heart health website, here are four of seven changes to make in your daily life to keep your heart healthy or make it healthy[12]:

------------------------

[12] *"7 Lifestyle Changes to Make After a Heart Attack." (2018, March 9). Retrieved from https://www.healthline.com/health/heart-disease/lifestyle-changes-after-heart-attack*

- **Up your food game**
  - » A healthy diet is one of the best ways to combat cardiovascular disease. You can begin by tracking how many calories you consume daily with a calorie counter app like *MyFitnessPal*. Determine how many calories you need in order to lose or maintain your weight, and stay within that range each day.
  - » Skip foods that have very few nutrients and a lot of calories. Limit saturated fat, trans fat, sodium, red meat, sweets, and sugar-sweetened beverages. Reduce or avoid processed foods (these are packed with sodium).
  - » Increase your vegetable and fruit intake. Include more whole grains, low-fat dairy products, lean proteins, and healthy oils.
- **Make a move**
  - » Cardiac rehabilitation is a great way to get started with exercise after a heart event. Exercise will help strengthen your heart and lowers your blood pressure and cholesterol levels. The American Heart Association recommends 150 minutes per week of moderate exercise, at least 75 minutes of vigorous exercise, or a combination of both.

● **Make the mind body connection**

  » Maintaining a positive attitude can benefit your health in many ways. If you have a positive outlook about your treatment after a heart attack, including any lifestyle changes, this can reduce your risk of heart problems.

  » After a heart attack, you'll likely experience a wide range of emotions, including depression and anxiety. These emotions can make it more difficult to implement and maintain habits that will greatly improve your health.

● **Maintain a healthy weight**

  » Carrying extra weight requires your heart to work harder, which in turn increases your risk of subsequent heart issues. If you have high blood pressure, high cholesterol, or high blood sugar, this can increase your risk even more. Introduce exercise and diet modifications into your life to lose weight and lower your risk factors.

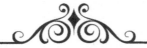

# CHAPTER EIGHT

# TAKING YOUR EMOTIONAL TEMPERATURE

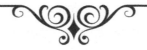

## Coping with Your Feelings

"The best and most beautiful things in the world cannot be seen
or even touched. They must be felt with the heart."
—Helen Keller

You're home. You might not be able to sleep or don't have much of an appetite. Maybe you feel alone or scared. You may, for the first time, grapple with your own mortality. Your moods may be on an emotional roller coaster. Not quite sure what to think about the future—when you'll return to work, drive, or if you'll ever have sex again. These feelings are common, and while it seems like they'll be around forever—they will not. As you learn how to manage heart disease, they will dissipate. Sometimes feelings, such as depression, may stay with you, in which case you should see a professional.

## Some Common Emotions

**Fear.** A heart attack is a traumatic event. It's normal to feel scared and uncertain about the future. We are often fearful because we have questions about how we'll manage. To ease your worry and fears:

- » Get answers to your questions. Prepare a list of questions for your doctor. Ensure you understand what to expect over the next several months and long-term.
- » Share with someone how you're feeling. Talk about how you feel with a family member, friend, your doctor, or counselor. Getting it out may help to comfort you.

**Anxiety.** Anxiety is a type of fear. It is your body's way of responding to stress. What makes you anxious? Pet and CT Scans, MRIs, and trips to the dentist make me very anxious. Anxiousness may show up as being nervous, tense, and irritable. To overcome anxiety:

» Reduce your caffeine intake. Caffeine gives us a jolt that may increase our energy. But, this nervous energy could cause an anxiety attack.

» Breathe. Deep breathing helps to calm you down. Focus on inhaling and exhaling deep breaths. This will help slow down and center your mind.

» Exercise. Engaging in exercise diverts you from what you're anxious about. Exercise is movement, and movement will decrease muscle tension, lowering the body's contribution to feeling anxious.

**Anger.** Heart attack patients often find themselves recovering both emotionally and physically. Learning that you have heart issues can be frustrating and distressing. Being angry is okay when it is expressed in a healthy way:

» Journal. For many people, anger includes impulsive outburst. Journaling about your angry feelings slows the entire anger process and gives you more time to deal with the feelings in an emotionally healthy way.

» Write a letter. When we are angry with someone, it may be difficult to express our anger without making the situation worse. And, it's not healthy to hold anger inside. A good way to deal with anger is to write a letter. Getting your thoughts and emotions out in the open will help you process in a positive way.

Be careful with this emotion. While it can be powerful if handled in a healthy way, it can be powerfully detrimental if you are frequently angry. Research from Harvard Medical School finds that frequent and extreme anger can cause your blood pressure and heart rate to increase, thus causing your heart to work harder. Research shows that in the two hours after an angry outburst, a person has a slightly higher risk of having chest pain (angina), a heart attack, a stroke, or a risky heart rhythm.

**Guilt.** This emotion fits very well into the conversation about anger. Could my heart event have been avoided? Long before my heart journey began, I remember a friend, Michelle, tell me, "My sister is okay. She *just* has to have another stent (absent of a heart attack). She keeps doing this (in reference to her sister's multiple stent placement). If she would just eat right and stop all of the bad eating."

According to the Heart and Stroke Foundation, there is a condition called *atherosclerosis*. Atherosclerosis occurs when your arteries become clogged with fatty deposits (plaque), causing them to lose elasticity and become narrower. Atherosclerosis is a slow, progressive condition that may begin as early as childhood. Its causes are complicated and not completely understood, but atherosclerosis is thought to start when the inner lining of the artery becomes damaged. [13]

If we eat all of the right foods, exercise religiously, and are at our most healthy weight, can we avoid heart disease or heart attack? I wish it were that easy. I talked with a fellow heart sister, Lana, who has been an exercise guru for many years. Absolutely no body fat. She had a heart attack.

Bob Harper, former host of the TV show *Biggest Loser*, was placed in a medically induced coma to give his heart some rest after he suffered a near-fatal heart attack. Prior to this life-changing event, he would have told you, "For me, having a heart attack is out of the question." According to an article on AARP.com, *"Biggest Loser* Host on His Heart Attack and Recovery," Bob Harper recalls signs like fainting during a workout. His doctor wanted to do further testing, but Bob put it off. Again, thinking there was no way a heart attack had his name on it, despite having lost both his mother and father to a heart attack.

--------------------

[13] *"Atherosclerosis: Also Called Hardening of Arteries." Retrieved from* https://www.heartandstroke.ca/heart-disease/conditions/atherosclerosis

Guilt should be a short-term emotion that you can channel into positive change. It's only a short-term emotion because long-term or chronic guilt is counterproductive and can lead to chronic illness. Chronic guilt can lead to anxiety, and anxiety can lead to stress causing illnesses. Feelings of guilt are absolutely normal. Let feelings of guilt propel you into making healthy lifestyle changes.

**Depression.** Are you like a lot of people—reluctant to admit depression? You are too blessed to be depressed or stressed, right? Why would you be depressed after surviving a heart attack? Statistics show you beat the odds. You could have died, but you didn't so you're lucky. Right? In their book *The Cancer Survivors Companion*, Dr. Frances Goodhart and Lucy Atkins explain this unspoken expectation can and often does backfire. They go on to say it can feel overwhelming and leave survivors feeling confused, lost, and low. There can be guilt and gloom right alongside the gratitude we feel for still being alive after surviving a life-threatening illness.[14]

---

[14] *Atkins, Lucy and Goodhart, Francis Dr. (2013). The Cancer Survivor's Companion: Practical Ways to Cope with Your Feelings after Cancer. Piatkus Publishing.*

A heart disease diagnosis or heart attack is overwhelming and can cause anxiety that may lead to depression. Think about it:

» Your life is put on hold for the length of time you are recovering and convalescing. This could be months and possibly years.

» The mortality issue rears its head making you think a lot about your death or the death of loved ones.

» You avoid anything that reminds you of the heart attack (for me I refused to travel to Detroit, and perhaps the worst was never eating again at an Arby's).

This is not something you should manage alone. Depression should be addressed in a healthy way. Share with your doctor and together come up with a plan of action.

According to the American Heart Association, one in ten Americans, age eighteen and older, have depression. Symptoms of depression are about three times more common in patients after an acute heart attack than in the general population, which strongly suggests a link between depression and heart disease.

While being diagnosed with heart disease or having a heart attack may increase the risk of depression, depression itself may increase the chances of developing heart disease. According to University of Iowa cardiologist Milena A. Gebska, M.D., Ph.D., "A number of factors may explain why patients with depression are at a higher risk for heart disease. There is a two-way relationship between heart disease and depression. On one hand, depression itself is an independent risk factor for adverse cardiac events in patients without known heart disease. On the other hand, patients with known heart disease, particularly those who develop a heart attack, are at increased risk of developing new diagnosis of depression."[15]

The following lifestyle changes can help manage both depression and heart disease:

» **Eat healthy foods:** A balanced diet will make you feel better, improve the health of your heart, and decrease your risk of heart disease.

» **Exercise regularly:** Exercise is a great form of therapy for people with depression and helps improve your heart health at the same time.

» **Drink less alcohol:** As a depressant, alcohol lowers the levels of serotonin (the chemical that regulates mood) in your brain. Hence, heavy alcohol consumption may

---

[15] *"Understanding the Link Between Depression and Heart Disease"* *(2016, January). Copyrighted material used with permission of the author, University of Iowa Hospitals & Clinics, uihc.org.*

cause your depression to worsen. Alcohol also increases the risk of high blood pressure, a major risk factor for heart attack or stroke. The American Heart Association recommends one to two drinks or less per day for men and one drink or less per day for women.

» **Quit smoking:** Many people who are depressed resort to smoking as a form of relaxation. Smoking is the number one preventable risk factor for developing heart disease. In other words, you can lower your chances of developing heart disease if you kick the habit. Talk with your doctor about healthier relaxation techniques.[16]

To help lower your stress, which may help with depression, try the following:

» Do deep breathing exercises.
» Use visualization (imagining beautiful settings, favorite memories).
» Get plenty of rest and sleep.
» Share your feelings with others or write them down.

------------------------

[16] *"Understanding the Link Between Depression and Heart Disease" (2016, January). Copyrighted material used with permission of the author, University of Iowa Hospitals & Clinics, uihc.org*

Again, seek out professional help to treat ongoing depression.

**Loneliness.** Difficult circumstances often bring people together. But following a heart attack, you may experience feelings of loneliness and isolation. You're the only one experiencing the effects the heart attack is having on you physically and emotionally. It's important to combat loneliness because it can cause further health issues. Here are some ways to overcome loneliness:

» Volunteer. Volunteering helps put the world in perspective. Start by giving a little time to a cause you care about. Not sure where to volunteer? Visit www.VolunteerMatch.com. Volunteering has been scientifically proven as a way to reduce stress.
» Read. If you like a good read, then you may enjoy being part of a book club. It can be fun and stimulating to discuss books with likeminded people.
» Join a heart support group. Heart support groups are friendly for people with heart conditions. Activities vary from outings to relevant talks about heart disease.

**Gratitude.** After a heart attack there is the obvious physical toll, but a heart event can also affect you mentally and emotionally. The initial relief you feel for having survived can be inundated by a myriad of emotions you didn't expect and don't know quite how to manage. One of the emotions that can help you after a heart attack is gratitude. Gratitude is a powerful emotion and one that can make your life better in so many ways. It is the habit and practice that may actually change your perception of well-being. "Gratitude is good medicine," says Robert A. Emmons, PhD., a professor of psychology at the University of California and author of *The Little Book of Gratitude*. "Clinical trials indicate that the practice of gratitude can have dramatic and lasting effects in a person's life. It can lower blood pressure and improve immune function. Grateful people engage in more exercise, have better dietary behaviors, are less likely to smoke and abuse alcohol, and have higher rates of medication adherence."[17]

**There are some simple ways to add gratitude to your life:**

- » Keep a gratitude journal and write in it daily.
- » Smile often.
- » Live mindfully for today—not worrying about the past or future.
- » Learn something new and be thankful.
- » Post positive quotes and images on social media.

------------------

[17] *American Heart Association News, "Gratitude is a Healthy Attitude."*

## Denise's Words of Wisdom (WOW)

**Your emotions will be all over the place.** Yes, they will. You may experience multiple emotions in a short period of time. You don't have to manage them alone. Please seek professional help if any of the emotions are lingering. Get support from people who have been where you are.

# Chapter Nine

# Bouncing Back
# After a Heart Attack

## Follow the Doctor's Orders

*"The comeback is always stronger than the setback."*
*—Unknown*

I f you've had a heart attack, you're probably wondering how your life is going to change. You might be feeling a little overwhelmed right now from hearing details of my heart journey, learning new medical information, and wondering what steps you can take towards recovery. Know that you are not alone. There are far too many people just like you who have thought about, or been rightfully concerned about, "What's next?"

As if the heart attack weren't shocking enough, the long list of to-dos from your doctor can seem daunting and come as a surprise. You may wonder "Everything on the list?" A study in the *Journal of the American Heart Association* shows how important it is to follow all of the doctor's orders. The study included more than 25,000 patients who had experienced heart attacks. After leaving the hospital, each person was given goals to work on. These goals were aimed at preventing another heart attack and improving survival. Over the next three months, the researchers checked in twice with the patients to see how well they followed recommendations. The researchers also tracked the patient's survival for up to four years afterward. They found that the more preventive steps people took, the more likely they were to survive. [18]

While I was in ICU, there were so many medicines I was given, including a Heparin shot twice a day. I didn't know I would have to still take medications when I got home. A lot of them that heart attack survivors are prescribed are *lifers* that we take forever. Early on I would forget to take my prescriptions and

---

[18] *"Heart Attack Patients Who Follow More Guidelines Live Longer."* *(2020, March 5). Retrieved from* https://www.eurekalert.org/pub_releases/2020-03/kp-hap030220.php

suffer the physical consequences. Remembering to take your medications can be very challenging, and remembering to take medications at multiple times of the day might feel overwhelming.

The medications we take can work wonders. However, in order to be effective you have to take all of your medications safely and as prescribed. Some best practices for maximum medication management:

1.  Be sure to make a list of every medication you take. List why you take it and what it looks like. Be prepared to ask your cardiologist why a particular medication has been prescribed. I have taken medication in the past and woke up with swollen eyes, vomited after putting eye drops in my eye, and developed a dry cough—all side effects of various medications.

2.  You'll need a plan for prescription replenishment. There are many options for getting our medications, including ordering them online or pharmacy pickup. The online ordering option is a great way to stock up, as most of these formats and some employer health plans require ordering prescriptions ninety days at a time.

3. When you have a doctor's appointment, take your prescriptions or a list of them with you. Even if your doctor prescribed them.

4. Invest in a pillbox or dispenser. A pill dispenser has a slot for each day of the week, and some even have a slot for morning, middle of the day, afternoon, and evening. Mine has the days of the week and holds one for morning and night. Be purposeful about planning out when you'll take your medication.

After a heart event, you may be prescribed some or all of the following medicines. You can read more about this on the website from The Society for Cardiovascular Angiography and Interventions.[19]

» **Antiplatelet agents**: Prevent blood clots and keep the stent open. Examples include aspirin, clopidogrel, prasugrel, and ticagrelor with brand names Plavix, Effient, and Brilinta respectively.

---

[19] *"Medications after a Heart Attack." (2014, November 12). Retrieved from https://www.secondcount.org/healthy-living/healthy-living-detail-2/medications-after-heart-attack#.X7QKEi2ZN-U*

» **Statins:** Lower cholesterol levels. Examples include atorvastatin by Lipitor, simvastatin made by Zocor, rosuvastatin by Crestor, or pravastatin by Pravachol.

» **Beta blockers**: Treat high blood pressure and decrease the incidence of abnormal heart rhythms. These also help the heart improve its function. In other words, the heart doesn't have to work as hard. Examples include metoprolol (Lopressor, Toprol XL), carvedilol (Coreg), nebivolol (Bystolic), atenolol (Tenomin), and bisoprolol (Zebeta).

» **ACE-inhibitors/Angiotensin receptor blockers (ARBs)**: Lower blood pressure. They can also help to improve heart function. ACE-inhibitors after large heart attacks have increased survival. Examples of ACE-inhibitors include lisinopril (Prinivil, Zestril), Ramipril (Altace), captopril (Capoten), quinapril (Accupril), and enalapril (Vasotec). Examples of ARBs include losartan (Cozaar), valsartan (Diovan), Irbesartan (Avapro), Olmesartan (Benicar), and azilsartan (Edarbi).

» **Calcium channel blockers**: Reduce blood pressure and control the amount of calcium that enters the heart and arteries, allowing blood vessels to relax and reduce the workload of the heart. An example is verapamil (Isoptin SR, Calan SR).

» **Nitrates**: Expand the arteries leading to the heart and relieve chest pain. Examples include sublingual nitroglycerin, isosorbide (Imdur), isosorbide dinitrate (Isordil), and the nitroglycerin patch. I wasn't prescribed nitroglycerin until years after my heart attack.

» **Antianginal agents**: Relieve chest pain. Besides nitrates (see above), ranolazine (Ranexa) may also be given to help decrease chest pain.

» **Anticoagulants**: Reduce the blood's ability to clot. If there is evidence of a blood clot in the heart after a heart attack, then warfarin (Coumadin) may be used to eventually dissolve the clot. If there is evidence for a certain type of abnormal heart rhythm, then depending on one's risk for stroke, warfarin (Coumadin), dabigatran (Pradaxa), or rivaroxaban (Xarelto) may be prescribed to thin the blood and decrease the risk for stroke.

Taking these medications may be new for you. It was for me. I had never taken anything except birth control pills. Take a deep breath and remember you're not alone. According to an article published in *Circulation*, the journal of the American Heart Association, "Heart attack patients who had not filled any of their prescriptions within 120 days of being discharged from the hospital had eighty percent greater odds of death than those who filled all of their prescriptions."[20]

After you've been on the medications for a while, talk to your cardiologist about when you can expect to come off of some of them. Most, if not all, heart attack survivors are advised to take a daily aspirin forever. If you received a bare metal stent, you should also take an antiplatelet (Plavix, Effient, or Brilinta) for a minimum of a month after the procedure. If you received a drug-eluting (coated) stent, you will have to take Plavix, Effient, or Brilinta for at least a year after stent implantation. A coated stent is a tiny cage used to keep a once clogged or blocked artery open and prevent it from closing again. The stent is coated with a drug. Taking these medications exactly as prescribed is critically important to preventing a blood clot from potentially forming in the stent.[21]

------------------------

[20] *"Medications after a Heart Attack." (2014, November 12). Retrieved from https://www.secondcount.org/healthy-living/healthy-living-detail-2/medications-after-heart-attack#.X7QKEi2ZN-U*

[21] *Shiel, Jr. MD, FACP, FACR, William C. "Medical Definition of Coated Stent." Retrieved from https://www.medicinenet.com/coated_stent/definition.htm*

Taking all of these medications are foreign to you and your body. You've just had a stressful event, and now you have a medication regimen. Antiplatelets can do a job on your stomach as well as increase the chance of bleeding from the stomach. Your cardiologist may recommend medications to protect the stomach. Examples include H2 blockers such as cimetidine (Tagamet), famotidine (Pepcid), and ranitidine (Zantac) or proton pump inhibitors such as pantoprazole (Protonix). Don't assume "If I needed it my doctor would prescribe it." Ask, "Do I need something for my stomach?" If the doctor says no, ask why not.

No one should have to remind you to take your prescriptions. Having a stroke or a subsequent heart attack should be reminder enough to do what's needed to live.

### Cardiac Rehabilitation.

Medication management is not the only order on the list. There were two decisions I was certain of when I was finally able to leave Michigan following the heart attack. 1) I would find a new cardiologist, and 2) I would go to cardiac rehabilitation (CR). Dr. Roger didn't give me a lot of details about it but told me it was mandatory that I attend cardiac rehab. I didn't realize it then but CR is underutilized, especially by women.

I met a fellow heart sister who didn't participate in CR. She said, "I was an avid exerciser before the *mishap*. I didn't have a heart attack and was stented once blockage was detected. I know how to exercise."

The purpose of CR is not to teach you how to exercise. It doesn't matter if you were exercising before your heart event. Following a heart attack or other heart event is not the time for a DIY (Do It Yourself) recovery plan. It's important to get help from an experienced expert.

Your cardiologist should prescribe cardiac rehabilitation. CR is about adopting a healthy lifestyle. The program includes exercise training, education on nutrition, and overall heart healthy living. It helps decrease the chances of you returning to the hospital with more heart issues. There is an entire cardiac rehab team including doctors, nurses, physical therapists, nutritionists, and counselors for mental health. You show up two to three times a week for 45-60 minutes. These sessions typically last two to three months. There are low-cost maintenance programs to help you after your initial sessions are over.

Cardiac rehab is covered by insurance and is not just for heart attack survivors. According to UnityPoint Health cardiologist Mohammand Saghir, MD, "In addition to the known cardiovascular benefits of exercise, cardiac rehab is associated with a 25% relative risk reduction in cardiovascular death and a 20% relative risk reduction in subsequent hospital admissions for heart issues." [22]

When you arrive for your cardiac rehab session, your blood pressure is taken. EKG leads are attached to you each and every time. Nurses and physical therapists literally monitor as you walk on the treadmill, ride the stationary bicycle, do resistance training, row on the rowing machine, and use the elliptical trainer.

After a heart attack, patients often have an understandable component of depression, anxiety, and fear to perform physical activity. Structured exercise in a monitored setting helps considerably to alleviate this concern. Following the heart attack, I was deathly afraid that I would do something, or nothing at all, and I would have another heart attack. Studies show "structured exercise" helps with the psychological and physical consequences of cardiac illness.

---

[22] *"Cardiac Rehabilitation: Exercising for Your Heart." (2015, July 25). Retrieved from https://www.unitypoint.org/article.aspx?id=711c3612-4a77-45d6-996b-d2ae51416a75*

**Driving Again.**

When can you get back behind the wheel after a heart attack? Typically, you'll have to wait at least two weeks, quite possibly longer, depending on a few factors. It depends on how you're progressing, the treatment you received, and the type of vehicle you want to drive. All of the driving particulars should be discussed with your doctor. The following are suggestions for wait time before driving:[23]

> » Cardiac arrest: at least six months.
> » Coronary artery bypass graft (CABG) surgery: at least four weeks.
> » Heart attack (myocardial infarction): at least two weeks.
> » Cardiac pacemaker: at least two weeks.
> » Coronary angiogram: at least two days.

Your doctor may give you clearance, but you may feel apprehensive. It's normal. Have a family member drive you or drive with you. Be sure to check with your car insurance carrier to see if there is a period time after your hospitalization that you are not covered.

------------------------------

[23] *"What Happens When I Get Home from the Hospital After a Heart Attack?" Retrieved from https://healthywa.wa.gov.au/Articles/U_Z/What-happens-when-I-get-home-from-hospital-after-a-heart-attack*

**Returning to Work.**

Getting back into the swing of things, including work, is an important part of your heart attack recovery. You might feel a little unsure about when you can go back and whether you'll be able to do the same kind of work. You can usually return to work within a few weeks or months after you leave the hospital. I returned to work on a part-time basis after about seven weeks. I continued on as part-time for about three months. Be sure to work with your human resources department regarding your return. There may be specific paperwork required for your return. Remember the following as you prepare to go back to work:

» Don't return too early. You may feel fit and great at home. Once at work you'll be required to give 100%.
» Be realistic. You will know when you're able to do something and when you don't feel up to it.
» Go back to a job you were already doing, if possible. Changing jobs, adding, or taking away responsibilities can be very stressful.

**Sex After a Heart Attack.**

It's not unusual for people to find that their health affects relationships. After a heart attack you may, like many other survivors, wonder whether it will be safe to resume sexual activity. You may worry about having another heart attack or dying during intimacy. Even though this is an incredibly necessary topic, people are often uncomfortable talking about it. The American Heart Association (AHA) commissioned a committee of experts in various fields to determine what is known on the topic. Some of the key points are[24]:

- **How stressful is sex on the heart?**
  - » Men and women have similar heart rate and blood pressure responses to sexual arousal. In young, healthy people, the physical demands of intercourse are equivalent to those of climbing two flights of stairs.

- **What is the risk of a heart attack during sex?**
  - » Less than 1% of all heart attacks occur during sexual activity. In men, the risk is as low for those who have suffered a heart attack as it is for those without coronary artery disease. A sedentary lifestyle increases the risk, but to a much greater extent in women than in men. The good news is

---

[24] *"Resuming Sex After a Heart Attack." (2012, August). Retrieved from https://www.health.harvard.edu/heart-health/resuming-sex-after-a-heart-attack*

that having sex regularly lowers the risk, likely by improving exercise capacity.

**Some guidelines when it comes to resuming intimacy:**
» If you've had surgery, wait until you're healed (usually 6-8 weeks). Don't put any weight on your chest.
» Avoid sex after eating a large meal, drinking alcohol, or when you're tired.

**Traveling by Plane.**
If you have flight travel plans, discuss them with your physician. Every airline will have a different procedure for travel after a heart attack. You may be advised, like I was, not to travel until you are stable.

» Airlines impose up to a ten-day waiting period for recent episodes of unstable angina (chest pain), myocardial infarction (heart attack), cardiac bypass surgery, acute heart failure, cardiac ablation, coronary stenting, or angiography (procedure that uses x-ray images to see heart).
» A good idea to obtain travel medical insurance that covers preexisting cardiac conditions.
» Have your medical history close by.

» Inform TSA of implanted defibrillators or pacemakers before going through screening.

### Denise's Words of Wisdom (WOW)

**Take your medication as prescribed.** There is no way around taking your medication. Taking prescriptions following a heart event are critical to your recovery and reduce the risk for future heart issues. As a suggestion, put a number on each prescription bottle matched to the number on your checklist. Check them off once they have been taken.

**Understand the medications you're taking.** It is completely natural to be concerned about side effects. Discuss any side effects with your cardiologist.

**Create a checklist.** For years to come, you will have to reference what kind of medication, how often, and how much you take. I got to the place I could spout off every prescription and dose. That's great, but what if you were incapacitated and couldn't remember or perhaps talk? It is a good idea to keep a checklist, and share it with a family member, with the following information:

» Name of prescriptions (both generic and brand name).

» What each medication is for.

» How much to take.

» How often to take.

» If they need to be taken at a certain time of day.

» If they interact with any foods or drinks.

» If they interact with any other medicine, you are taking.

**Cardiac Rehabilitation is necessary.** Cardiac rehab is as necessary as taking prescribed medication is to your overall heart recovery. It is one of the best things you can do for yourself—start and complete your program.

**Previous exercise is not a prerequisite.** Whether I was an exerciser or not is irrelevant when it comes to cardiac rehabilitation. Everyone is monitored. No one comes in and does their own exercise plan.

**Returning to work.** Most heart attack patients go back to work within two weeks to three months depending on the severity of the heart attack. Your doctor will determine when you can go back and if your current job is suitable for a person who has had a heart attack.

**Sex and intimacy.** You may feel less interested or able for a while. This is normal. Be patient until things get back to normal.

*I Don't Want to Die Like This*

**Travel by plane.** Always let your doctor know about your travel plans. When traveling, particularly overseas, purchase travel insurance that includes a preexisting condition.

100

# Chapter Ten
# Under New Management

## *Managing Risk Factors*

They call them risk factors. Post heart event, we have to manage them. If you haven't had a heart event, there are ways to lower your risk for heart disease. Some of the risk factors we have no control over such as increasing age, gender, and heredity. The majority of people who die as a result of heart disease are over the age of sixty-five. According to statistics, men are more apt to have a heart attack. African Americans have a greater chance of having high blood pressure. Heart disease is also higher among Mexican Americans, American Indians, native Hawaiians, and some Asians. According to the American Heart Association, this is due partly to higher rates of obesity and diabetes.[25]

But, there is good news. There are risk factors that you can change and control.

**Smoking**. Not much to say except if you smoke, you are at a much higher risk of developing heart disease, stroke, or having a heart attack. Smoking is also a risk for cardiac arrest. Second hand smoke is a contributing factor to heart disease for nonsmokers. Talk with your healthcare provider for help in finding the best way for you to quit. Also, limit alcohol consumption. Drinking too much alcohol can cause your blood pressure to increase.

**High blood cholesterol**. Gosh, that sounds like when your mom used to call you by your entire name. You knew something was awry, didn't you? When it comes to your high blood cholesterol, if it is increasing, so is your risk for coronary heart disease. If you have had a heart event, then your risks for having another one goes up right along with your cholesterol.

---

[25] *"Understand Your Risks to Prevent a Heart Attack." Retrieved from https://www.heart.org/en/health-topics/heart-attack/understand-your-risks-to-prevent-a-heart-attack*

I recently went in for my annual exam with Dr. Beta. She was reviewing my blood work. She told me all of the good numbers and then with a sense of urgency shared, "Your low-density-lipoprotein is extremely high." Say what now? My LDL (bad cholesterol) was too high. She said, "The numbers are high for anyone but particularly concerning for someone with your history of heart disease." She put me on Atorvastatin again and shared that a Mediterranean diet would help as well.

**Let's break down high blood cholesterol[26]:**

&raquo; **Total cholesterol.** This is your total cholesterol and is calculated using the following: HDL (see below for explanation) + LDL + 20 percent of your triglyceride level. I know the terms may be foreign...but stay with me.

&raquo; **Low-density-lipoprotein (LDL) cholesterol** = bad cholesterol. An LDL cholesterol level is considered good for your heart health. Making lifestyle changes to your diet, such as lowering your intake of high saturated and trans fats, can have a positive impact on your LDL.

---

[26] *"HDL (Good), LDL (Bad) Cholesterol and Triglycerides." Retrieved from https://www.heart.org/en/health-topics/heart-attack/understand-your-risks-to-prevent-a-heart-attack*

» **High-density-lipoprotein (HDL) cholesterol** = good cholesterol. The higher this number the better for your heart health. The lower the number the higher the risk for heart disease. Genetic factors such as Type 2 diabetes, smoking, and being overweight negatively impact this number. Also, being sedentary lowers this number.

» **Triglycerides.** These are the most common type of fat in the body. Normal triglyceride levels vary by age and sex. A high triglyceride level combined with low HDL or high LDL is associated with atherosclerosis, which is the buildup of fatty deposits inside artery walls that increase the risk for a heart attack and stroke.

**High blood pressure.** If you're new to high blood pressure, you might feel overwhelmed and/or worried about what having high blood pressure means. High blood pressure increases the heart's workload, which makes the heart muscle thick and become stiff. Stiffening of the heart muscle is not normal and thus causes the heart to function abnormally. Having high blood pressure increases your risk of stroke, heart attack, kidney failure, and congestive heart failure.

Buy a blood pressure monitor. Now that you've had a heart event, at some point your cardiologist is going to ask you to track your blood pressure...or heck, you want to know your own numbers. There is a right and a wrong way to take your blood pressure. Be still. Don't smoke, drink caffeinated beverages, or exercise thirty minutes before measuring your blood pressure. Doctors advise you should empty your bladder and have a full five minutes of quiet rest before taking the measurements. Sit straight up (hard back chair) vs. a bed or couch. Feet should be flat on the floor, and do not cross your legs. Why? Crossing one leg over the other causes a temporary spike in the blood pressure. You should take the measurements at the same time every day and record the numbers.

Put down the salt. If that sounded a little harsh, it's not you...it's me. I have struggled with salt for a very long time. There are some great substitutes out there including Mrs. Dash. And, did you know Mrs. Dash comes in different flavors? Read the labels on your food. Watch the sodium intake as well as stay away from processed foods as much as possible. Processed foods have a lot of sodium. Potassium can lower the effects of sodium on blood pressure. The best sources of potassium come from fruits and vegetables.[27]

Find ways to reduce your stress and lower the risk for heart disease. Easier said than done, right? Chronic stress may contribute to high blood pressure. Really think about what causes you stress. For me? Trips to the grocery store. I loathe being inside them. I manage the stress by avoidance. Mom does all of the grocery shopping (she loves it). The few times I was in charge of pantry replenishment, I ordered the groceries and had them delivered. Extreme stress can be a "trigger" for a heart attack. Some common ways to manage stress include overeating, smoking, and heavy drinking—all of which are bad for your heart. Manage stress by exercising or do something calming like deep breathing, gardening, reading, or meditating.

Diabetes. Having diabetes means you are more likely to develop heart disease, which of course means you are at greater risk for a heart attack or stroke. The best way to manage diabetes and protect your heart is to control your blood glucose, which is also referred to as blood sugar, blood pressure, and

------------------

[27] *"Understanding the Heart-healthy Benefits of Potassium."*
*Retrieved from https://www.heart.org/en/health-topics/high-blood-pressure/changes-you-can-make-to-manage-high-blood-pressure/how-potassium-can-help-control-high-blood-pressure*

cholesterol. What do the readings mean? Report unusually high and low blood pressure readings to your doctor. Share with your doctor what's working and what's not working when it comes to your blood pressure medication. [28]

| BLOOD PRESSURE CATEGORY | SYSTOLIC mm Hg (upper number) | | DIASTOLIC mm Hg (lower number) |
|---|---|---|---|
| NORMAL | LESS THAN 120 | and | LESS THAN 80 |
| ELEVATED | 120 – 129 | and | LESS THAN 80 |
| HIGH BLOOD PRESSURE (HYPERTENSION) STAGE 1 | 130 – 139 | or | 80 – 89 |
| HIGH BLOOD PRESSURE (HYPERTENSION) STAGE 2 | 140 OR HIGHER | or | 90 OR HIGHER |
| HYPERTENSIVE CRISIS (consult your doctor immediately) | HIGHER THAN 180 | and/or | HIGHER THAN 120 |

Being physically inactive is a risk factor that we can control. Regular physical activity helps reduce the risk of cardiovascular disease. There are so many benefits of physical activity including controlling cholesterol, diabetes, and obesity. And, it plays a part in lowering blood pressure.

---

[28] *"Diastole vs. Systole: Know Your Blood Pressure Numbers." Retrieved from* https://www.webmd.com/hypertension-high-blood-pressure/guide/diastolic-and-systolic-blood-pressure-know-your-numbers#1

When we're overweight, especially around the mid-section, it makes us more susceptible to heart disease. "You mean I have to recover from a heart attack and lose weight?" Yes, but don't let losing weight overwhelm you. Literally, take it one day at a time. Set out to take the right steps every day. To lose weight the first step is set realistic goals. Know and understand your body mass index. Start off with small changes. Participating in cardiac rehab is a great boost for making changes in your lifestyle. I've always found when I record what I eat, (yes, write everything down that goes in your mouth), I lose weight. Manage your portion sizes. The portion sizes we get in restaurants are not an exercise in portion control. You can manage risks by being physically active—challenge yourself to walk another 150 more steps each day. Try to limit saturated fats, foods high in sodium, and added sugars. Eat plenty of fresh fruit, vegetables, and whole grains.

Sleeping. Getting enough sleep is important. Believe it or not, if you don't get enough sleep, it puts you at risk for raised blood pressure, being overweight, and diabetes. All three of these factors increase the risk for heart disease or another heart attack. Most adults need between seven to nine hours of sleep every night. Frequent sleep problems might be a sign of sleep apnea. Sleep apnea causes people to briefly stop breathing multiple times during the night.[29] As you can imagine, this disrupts your sleep and subsequently raises your risk for heart disease. Talk with your doctor about conducting a sleep study.

### Denise's Words of Wisdom (WOW)

**Every area of your life has to be on point.** Your diet has to be such that your blood pressure is controlled, diabetes is managed, waistline is diminishing—all while getting enough sleep. Yes, it can seem overwhelming. One day at a time.

**Losing weight.** Be sure your efforts at losing weight are natural. Stay away from diet pills. They increase your risk for heart attack and stroke. There may be diet pills safe for people with heart disease—you'll need to discuss with your doctor.

**Sleep.** Snoring doesn't automatically mean you suffer from sleep apnea; however, it is a good indicator. If you think you may have sleep apnea, discuss going through a sleep study to confirm. These are expensive. Your doctor may be called upon to make a case and explain to your medical insurance provider to get the study approved. Be patient if the test is initially denied.

---

[29] *"Sleep Apnea." Retrieved from https://www.mayoclinic.org/diseases-conditions/sleep-apnea/symptoms-causes/syc-20377631*

# CHAPTER ELEVEN
# OTIS D. POWELL

## Finding a Support System

*"People don't always need advice. Sometimes all they really
need is a hand to hold, an ear to listen,
and a heart to understand them."*
*—Zig Ziglar*

A couple of years after I got married, my then husband Ronald talked about getting a dog. I was very clear—NO DOG. I just wasn't much of an animal person.

Just for fun I asked, "What kind of dog would you want if I agreed to get a dog?" He said, "An English Bulldog." I was dismissive when I replied, "I don't even know what an English Bulldog looks like." He found a picture. I took one look at it and proclaimed loudly, "That is the ugliest dog I have ever seen!" With that the subject was closed.

I was thirty-four years old when I had a miscarriage. I moped around the house for days. I knew the chances of me having a baby were slim. I could have used a support group. Instead, one day Ronald came home and asked me to take a ride with him. I looked a mess and felt depressed but went on the ride. When we arrived at the house, he invited me to get out of the car. Barreling towards me was an ugly dog. A guy at the door said, "She just wants to smell you." As we walked in, I noticed a baby playpen but not a human baby in sight. Instead, there were two of the most adorable bulldog puppies looking at me. My heart started to melt.

Bill, the guy who I now know was the breeder, picked up the cutest one and put him in my arms. Oh, my goodness...I was in love. With a big smile Bill asked me, "What will you name him? I said firmly, "We're not naming him anything because we're not taking him." All the while I fell deeper and deeper in love with the puppy's eyes. I asked, "Out of curiosity, how much is he?" "1,500." I replied, "Dollars?" I politely handed that adorable puppy back to Bill and we left.

Three days later Bill called. When I said, "I'll let my husband know you called," he replied, "I just want you to know Ronald told me about your miscarriage. I'm so sorry and I would like to drop the price to $1,000." I smiled and said, "Thank you, I'll let him know."

Ronald came in grinning from ear to ear with all kinds of toys and a big crate. "Come on, let's go get Otis!" When we arrived, Ronald was preparing the crate for Otis and Bill said, "I don't think he's getting in the crate." Otis rode all the way back home on my lap. It took him a couple of nights to settle in, and I slept on the floor near him. He became my baby and was my therapy. Much to Ronald's chagrin I bought Otis sweaters, cooked him chicken breast, and just spoiled him.

Fast forward to May 2007. Ronald and I had separated, and while I was visiting a friend, Otis overheated. We drove to the nearest veterinary hospital, and the vet staff rushed out to get him...Otis was already gone. I was devastated.

Even though cremation was an expensive option, I wanted that for Otis. It would help me recover from the loss. Mom arrived and I was in no shape to drive. All I wanted to do was go to bed. I cried for days. People found out and I received cards, phone calls, and a couple of gift cards. I didn't even know there were pet/sympathy cards.

Every person who sent me a card and most who checked on me had experienced the loss of a pet. There is nothing more comforting, calming, and reassuring to me than someone who understands by experience. Maybe that's why my heart sisters are special to me. Even though our stories are different, we share a common understanding through experience.

A traumatic health event like a heart attack can have devastating emotional and physical effects on you. Many people who have experienced a heart attack put all of their focus on recovering physically, while they ignore their mental health needs. I can't emphasize enough how important a support group is to your recovery.

It is imperative that following a heart event you surround yourself with people who care as well as people who understand what you've gone through. Holding my hand, listening, and empathy was how I made it after Otis died. I didn't think I would.

After the heart attack I didn't realize I needed anyone besides my mom. She flew from Dallas to Indiana then on to Detroit. She got there and never left my side. There are times when, five years later, my seventy-seven year old mom will remark, "That's too heavy for you to lift." It's my mom who brings me tea every morning. She's my caregiver and confidant. Yet no matter how much I try to explain what happened, she doesn't fully know what it was like because she's never had a traumatic physical heart event. Her experience has been emotional, and she can support me from a caring, loving heart.

There is a support organization for every type of vice you can think of—sex addicts, gamblers, alcoholics and children of alcoholics, drug users, mothers against drunk drivers, cancer survivors, and so many others. Doesn't it make sense we would have one too?

My support came from the women in WomenHeart.[30] This group is the first and only national patient-centered organization dedicated to serving women with heart disease. WomenHeart believes education, support, and training enable women to take charge of their heart health and advocate for other women. I met a fellow heart sister at cardiac rehab. We joined our local WomenHeart group at the same time and attended our first meeting together. I was delighted to know that crying is normal. My theme song could be "It's my *body* and I'll cry if I want too."

All of us in the group have experienced some kind of heart event. From stent placement preventing a heart attack, to valve replacement, to heart transplants. We meet at least once a

---

[30] *https://www.womenheart.org/findsupport/*

month. We cry, sometimes. We always support each other, learn, and have fun.

WomenHeart hosts an annual WomenHeart Champion symposium. It's three days of networking, learning, and having a good time with fellow heart event survivors. I went in 2017 and saw women from the age of twenty-two to late seventies. Every woman had a different heart story. We learned how to harness our story into a concise, comprehensive opportunity to teach and inform every time we share it.

There are a number of organizations that provide support for women, men, and children. I have listed a few below, and I encourage you to find a local group that is right for you. The American Heart Association is the most recognized name in heart health. I love them and what they stand for. Although their focus isn't as a support group for individuals, they are dedicated to improving heart health and reducing deaths from cardiovascular diseases and stroke. Their website includes information such as scientific research, heart attack and stroke symptoms, heart healthy recipes, and numerous health articles. They are also the foremost authority on CPR (Cardiopulmonary resuscitation).

Support is a vital component to your recovery, and participating in a support group has many benefits including:

» Enhanced quality of life.

» Improved ability to communicate with your healthcare provider and family members.

» An increased understanding of heart disease.

» Increased ability to manage your treatment/medication regimen.

» A greater adherence to lifestyle changes to improve your health.

Sometimes we don't even realize we need support until we're being supported. Support can show up in the most unlikely of places and people. However, it shows up, gratefully take it all in and use what's best for your own recovery.

### Denise's Words of Wisdom (WOW)

**Talk to someone who understands.** There are support groups for everything you or someone you know are going through, have already experienced, or may face in the future. Whether it's losing a beloved pet or a heart attack, support can be very therapeutic.

A list of some heart related support groups and organizations:

» Adult Congenital Heart Association (ACHA)

» American Heart Association

- American Stroke Association
- Aortic Hope
- Ben's Friends
- Canadian Adult Congenital Heart Network
- The Children's Heart Foundation
- Children's Heart Network
- Cleveland Clinic Stroke and Brain Aneurysm Support Group
- CongenitalHeartDefects.com
- Congenital Heart Information Network
- Congenital Heart Surgeon's Society
- Conquering CHD
- Mended Hearts
- WomenHeart

**Don't see what you need?** Maybe the right group for you isn't listed. If you search the Internet and still don't see it, perhaps it's time for you to help create it.

**Journal.** Sometimes there are feelings and thoughts you want to say but can't or are afraid to. Writing down what's on your mind does amazing things for your mental, physical, and spiritual health. I have found journaling helps to prioritize problems, fears, and concerns. My health has improved, in part, because of journaling. When I journal, it helps to relieve stress.

It is calming—I know that my blood pressure stays within normal range because I journal every day.

There are both short and long-term benefits of journaling including stress relief. "Journaling is an incredible stress management tool, a good-for-you habit that lessens impact of physical stressors on your health. In fact, a study showed that expressive writing (like journaling) for only fifteen to twenty minutes a day, three to five times over the course of a four-month period, was enough to lower blood pressure and improve liver functionality."[31]

---------------------
[31] *"5 Powerful Health Benefits of Journaling." (2018, July 31).*
*Retrieved from*
*https://intermountainhealthcare.org/blogs/topics/live-well/2018/07/5-powerful-health-benefits-of-journaling/*

# CHAPTER TWELVE

# WHEN YOUR CHEST HURTS (AFTER A HEART ATTACK)

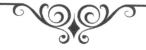

## Understanding Second Heart Attacks

*"Although the world is full of suffering,*
*it is full also of the overcoming of it."*
*—Helen Keller*

I s chest pain normal after a heart attack? Once you've had a heart attack, you're at a higher risk of having another one. One thing is for sure...after surviving a heart attack, you don't want another one. Yet, about one in five people who have had a heart attack will be readmitted to the hospital for a second one within five years. Each year there are about 335,000 recurrent heart attacks in the United States. [32]

It had been about ten days since the heart attack. Mom and I were at a hotel. She had been taking care of me nonstop and was tuckered out. I was unbelievably tired and moved at a snail's pace.

Acutely aware of everything that happened with my heart, I sat up when I felt something now familiar—chest pain. It's interesting that I used to only think about my heart when a doctor had the stethoscope and said, "Take a deep breath." Now I'm constantly aware.

Heart attack survivor hear me...from now on whenever you have an ailment, your caregiver and people close to you will ask, "Is it your heart?" It's true they are concerned and will want to know, "Does it feel like when you had the heart attack?" Your doctor will want you to describe the pain, too.

I rubbed my chest and the pain wasn't going away. If only it were that easy. I gently touched Mom. She woke up with a

---

[32] *"Proactive Steps Can Reduce Chances of Second Heart Attack." (2019, April 4). Retrieved from* https://www.heart.org/en/news/2019/04/04/proactive-steps-can-reduce-chances-of-second-heart-attack

startle. I told her about the chest pain. I described the pain as a two on a scale of zero to ten, and we took a risk and decided to forego the ambulance and called Uber. We got caught in a traffic jam and fortunately arrived at the hospital without any increase in my pain level.

It was a busy Thursday night in ER, and they took me right away at the mention of chest pain. They moved even quicker when I shared about the prior heart attack. They did an EKG, and it showed the heart attack. An EKG can tell if you've had a heart attack in the past. The staff felt confident I wasn't having another heart attack, BUT they didn't feel comfortable to let me go home. That night they kept me for observations.

In the years following my heart attack, we made a few trips to ER. Why? You don't ever want to feel like you did when you had the heart attack or heart event and risk your life. One of those times was October 5, 2019. Mom and I had been running errands all day, and we stopped for dinner. I tend to eat a little fast and thought I was having indigestion on our ride home. Heart attack pain for me was a twenty on a scale of zero to ten, and this was a seven. In retrospect, I made a mistake in judgment and should have gone straight to the nearby hospital or called an ambulance.

We weren't far from home, and when we got there I went to straight to my room and laid down on the bed. Our motto is, "If hot tea can't fix it, things are bad." Mom brought me tea, and I couldn't drink it. I put a tablet of my nitroglycerin prescription under my tongue, but it didn't help. By now it had been twenty minutes since the pain started. Mom wisely called 911, and the ambulance arrived. The paramedics checked my vitals and although they looked good, the guys suggested I go to the hospital as a precaution. I climbed on the gurney myself and waited for them to pull away. My heart rate began to drop, they got it back up, and took off to the hospital.

ER was packed, they put me in a room, and as I waited suddenly became really hot. Mom stood on one side of the bed, a nurse on the other, and they started to fan me. Abruptly, I turned to my mom and said, "I'm going to pass out." The last thing I heard was the nurse say, "Keep fanning her" and she took off running. When I later opened my eyes, there were several medical staff in the room, and on my chest and back were external defibrillator pads...a medical device to reset or restart the heart. I had become unresponsive.

I now have a pacemaker as a result of that experience. After a heart attack, you will feel pain, and sometimes it is just indigestion. On other occasions, like my situation, it really is something medically going on that requires attention. According to statistics, every 2.63 minutes a survivor has another heart attack. Within five years of a first heart attack, one in five survivors will have a second heart attack or die from one.[33] I share this not to be overly dramatic or frighten you but to stress that sometimes you need medical attention. Don't take any chances with your heart. Even if you feel as though you know how to distinguish one kind of chest pain from another. I learned my heart health lessons the hard way and want to help you, or someone you care about, with the knowledge and experience I gained.

Chest pain comes in many forms. The pain can range from a sharp stab to a dull ache. Sometimes it feels crushing or burning. Examples of heart-related causes of chest pain include:

» **Angina.** Angina is the term for chest pain caused by poor blood flow to the heart.
» **Aortic dissection.** This life-threatening condition involves the main artery leading from your heart (aorta).

---

[33] *"Celebrating Stories of Heart Survivorship." Retrieved from* https://www.survivorshaveheart.com/

» **Coronary Artery Spasms.** A temporary tightening (constriction) of the muscles in the wall of one of the arteries that send blood to your heart.

» **Pericarditis.** This is the inflammation of the sac surrounding your heart. It usually causes sharp pain that gets worse when you breathe in or when you lie down.

If you have new or unexplained chest pain or suspect you're having a heart attack—even when the pain is different from before—call for emergency help immediately. Many people think hopping in a car is faster and cheaper, but calling an ambulance when it matters could save a life.

### Denise's Words of Wisdom (WOW)

**Think about your heart.** Before my heart attack in 2015, I never gave thought to my heart. Maybe you were the same way. Now you may find yourself thinking about it all the time. You know your body better than any doctor. If it doesn't feel right to you, seek medical attention.

**Take an ambulance.** I said this in an earlier chapter. The only time you should have someone other than a paramedic drive you to the emergency room is if you are way up in the mountains and there is no phone service to call for an ambulance.

Seriously! If a paramedic can't get you there faster than a car, they can call ahead and have the ER team waiting on you.

**Nitroglycerin.**[34] What is it? It is a vasodilator, which is a medicine that opens blood vessels to improve blood flow. It is used to treat angina (chest pain or pressure) symptoms that happen when there is not enough blood flowing to the heart. It should reduce the chest pain. If the pain doesn't subside or gets worse after five minutes, you should call 911.

Not all cardiologists prescribe nitroglycerin. They have their reasons. If they don't prescribe it to take as needed, ask why not.

---

[34] *"Using Nitroglycerin for Angina." Retrieved from*
*https://www.uofmhealth.org/health-library/hw85228spec#*

# Part Three
# Balance and Bliss

# CHAPTER THIRTEEN

# WHODNI

## Finding Support through Friendships

*"True love and loyal friends*
*are two of the hardest things to find."*
*—Anonymous*

I n 1984 hip-hop group Whodini released their song "Friends." The chorus says, "Friends, how many of us have them, friends the ones you can depend on." Going through a major trauma like a heart attack had this song swarming around in my head for weeks. This was by far the most difficult chapter to write because of the emotions I felt remembering back to the initial event and following months of challenging recovery.

Did you ever have to come face to face with the fact that people who you thought would show up for you...didn't? Or they did but on their timeline or conditions? I didn't see this phase of my recovery coming, and I was blindsided by the hurtful reality of life.

Friendships are some of the most enduring and amazing gifts of life. Our first encounter with friendship likely came about without much effort because we met a childhood friend playing, shared a toy, and had fun. As time goes by, some of our friendships develop into meaningful exchanges of support, companionship, and whatever we need. Until they don't. There is no way to know the friendship tipping point...that event that causes a relationship to change. It might be a move, marriage, divorce, or in my case massive heart attack.

There is a quote that says, *"We never lose friends. We simply learn who the real ones are."* You find out who your real ones are after a heart event. Friendships change throughout your life, and people will surprise you. Unfortunately, people who have been a "friend" start showing up far differently than you ever expected...or not showing up at all. The same applies to family members. I don't mean just physically being with you. During your recovery you will need people to be there for you emotionally, spiritually, supportively, and physically. Some friends will be with you in all four ways and others just one.

Whatever it is, embrace and appreciate those important friends and family who do.

I've told you about my mother, best friend Terri and husband Paul, cousin Terrie, and co-worker Carlos who were the first family and friends to support me. There were several others, and some who didn't know what to say but showed they cared in various ways. My heart sisters have become a huge part of my support system.

I could write about the friends and family who never called, visited, or made excuses not to show up, but I have chosen not to. I experienced a lot of hurt and anger. My expectations were shattered. Some of those feelings came back as I wrote this book. Just like physical recovery is an ongoing process, so is emotional and spiritual. There has been so much written about the effects of a negative mindset on our physical bodies. I continue to work on my feelings and how to express them, and I have changed my unrealistic expectations of others and myself. I choose to live in a healthier way for myself and those relationships close to me and ones I can impact with my message of preventative health and how to recover and thrive after a major heart event.

Another surprise to me was if your recovery takes longer than people think it should, they begin to share stories of heart attack triumphs. For example, someone will undoubtedly tell you about a person who had a heart attack and went back to work in less than a month. Carlos was gentle but quick to set me straight on my unrealistic expectation of being back in the office. I heard about a guy who ran a marathon a month after he had a heart attack. Prepare for the story about the person who had the widow-maker, and they didn't even know they were having a heart attack. I found it best not to go into defense mode. People often don't know what to say and think their stories are helpful. You don't need a set of statistics to support where you are on your heart journey. It's your recovery, and you don't have to justify anything to anyone.

I have a friend who was diagnosed with breast cancer years ago. I literally stopped what I was doing and went to be with her. I never missed a chemo appointment and created a meal train. Years later when she wanted to celebrate five years cancer free, I flew home. She never had to wonder about my friendship. I tell this not to say, "Look at me! I'm such a good friend" but to let you know there are people who will support you like crazy, often because they know what it feels like. I certainly do. There are others who simply enjoy giving because that's how God made them. I may not be the first to volunteer to watch your kids, but I'll definitely bring over a hot meal, listen to you, and enjoy a good laugh if you need one.

Friends will come and go in your life. Simon Sinek, one of my favorite motivational speakers said, "The strong bond of friendship is not always a balanced equation...instead friendship is grounded in feeling that you know exactly who will be there for you when you need something no matter what or when." Maybe you've never evaluated your friendships or felt like it was necessary. A chapter on friendship is not here by accident. In order to have balance and bliss following a heart event, you have to understand the nature of your friendships. It will become clear who is there for you and what to do when others are not.

Years after the heart attack, I was having the first gala for the nonprofit I founded, *Fresh Start for Your Heart.* https://www.freshstartheart.org. I had been online talking about the event. At the event I looked up and saw a good friend I worked with at State Farm. Lisa and I met working together on an ice, snow, and sleet catastrophe. We became quick friends. I was in her wedding and she was in mine. I flew to Georgia when she had her first child. Lisa flew to Texas for those two hours of the gala event. She didn't even have time to come to the house afterwards, but Lisa was there to celebrate with me. As I write about this memory...our friendship makes me cry happy tears.

**Denise's Words of Wisdom (WOW)**

**Just what you need.** I am a firm believer God will put who you need in your life when they need to be there.

**Support.** Your support may not come from the friendships you've always known. Adjust your expectations in case support comes from an unlikely source.

# Chapter Fourteen
# Getting Your
# House in Order

## Compile, Gather, and Organize Important Papers

*"Getting your house in order and reducing the confusion gives you more control over your life. Personal organization somehow releases or frees you to operate more effectively."*
—Larry King

O ne of the best ways to demonstrate your love for your family and friends is to follow all of the doctor's orders, manage risks, and get your house in order. You're reading this book that indicates you either have suffered a heart attack, had some other heart event, you have a loved one who has suffered a heart attack, or you're being proactive.

You now have an opportunity to get your house in order. When I looked up "getting your house in order" it means *to improve or correct the way one does things*. The website Takebackyourtemple.com says getting one's house in order could mean many things from relating to your physical house, your finances, your family, or your health.

Five months before one of my best friends Tammy died, she sent me and two other friends an email with "My Wishes" in the subject line. She said, "The tone of this letter is not to be sad or a prophesy of my imminent death." She wanted us to know her final wishes in light of everything she had going on. Tammy had been battling cancer for years and was planning to divorce her husband. When we got the email, the cancer had spread to her brain, lungs, and so many other body parts. In her email she was clear about everything from repast to her remains.

In March of 2017, I got a phone call. I didn't recognize the number, so I let it go to voicemail. I realized the number had the same prefix as Tammy's and thought, "She must be calling me from a different number, or maybe she has a new number." I quickly called the number back, and it was her husband. He calmly told me, "Tammy isn't doing well." My mind raced—Tammy had beaten cancer too many times to count. I responded, "I will get a flight and be there by the weekend." There was so much silence I thought I had lost him and said,

"Hello?" He cleared his throat and said, "Okay, but she is going into hospice. We're just waiting on a bed." There was no way to soften that blow. I said, "I will be there in two days." I hung up and cried.

Support and communication is so important during a health crisis. The next day I received a call from Tammy's best friend Jolene. She said, "The doctor just left Tammy's room and doesn't believe she will make it through the night." From that moment, I don't remember a lot. I immediately changed my ticket and took Uber to the airport. I was a basket case. I desperately wanted to say goodbye to my friend. My bestie, Terri, was waiting to take me to the hospital. She gave me the keys instead and said, "Drive to my house when you're finished."

I made it to Tammy's room and sat next to her bed talking with her. I told her, "Thank you for waiting for me. I want you to know you've done a fabulous job raising two amazing kids. It's okay for you to go—we will miss you terribly and love you forever. We will all be okay.

Tammy had known for a while the end of life was coming soon. Two months before she sent the "My Wishes" email, she told me, "The cancer has spread to my brain among other places." When I asked her about us having a girls' weekend, she didn't say no. Every new tumor I always asked the same question, "Should I come home for a just us girls' weekend?" This time she said, "Yes." I should have known the time was soon. Tammy took trips with the kids—together and individually with both of them. She was slaying it at work. Moving and shaking. She had time to get her house in order and she did.

Two things are certain—taxes and death. We know when it's tax day but never really know when death will happen. How is your house? Is it in order? Gosh, if I hadn't survived the heart attack, I'm here to tell you my house wasn't in order. Mom didn't know my passwords, anything about my finances, or final wishes.

Your family should have all of this information. Here are some steps to take towards getting your house in order:

> » Gather and organize important documents in one place, including birth certificates, trusts, mortgage, power of attorney, etc. Secure hard copies in a fire and burglar proof safe. Soft copies should be password protected. Be sure to backup anything stored on your computer.
> » Compile financial documents—your investments and assets. Meet with your financial planner to ensure your will or trust is updated.

» Be just as concerned with your end of life and healthcare directives. This includes a living will, Health Insurance Portability and Accountability waiver (this allows doctors to give your healthcare information to third parties, including your family), and how you want your organs disposed.

» Provide details of your final wishes. Don't make family guess what you would have wanted.

» Create a legacy statement. It leaves a record of what you hope to pass on to the next generation.

A fatal heart attack doesn't give you a chance to get things in order. Getting your house in order is the best gift you can give your family.

# CHAPTER FIFTEEN
# TAKE CARE OF YOU!

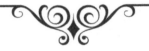

## Be an Advocate for Yourself

E very forty seconds someone has a heart attack. Every eighty seconds someone dies from heart disease. Ninety percent of women have at least one risk factor for heart disease and are less likely to survive their first heart attack.[35] What would you do if you noticed chest pain, shortness of breath, or dizziness? Would you call 911 or brush it off?

---

[35] *"Be Your Own Advocate: Speak Up for Your Heart Health."* Retrieved from *https://www.wellaheadphilly.com/introducing-well-ahead-philly-be-your-own-advocate-speak-up-for-your-heart-health/*

Despite increased awareness about heart disease, many women—and even some doctors—still dismiss or misdiagnose its symptoms as stress or anxiety. A study confirms fifty-three percent of young women with heart attack symptoms said that their health care provider did not think symptoms like stomach pain, shortness of breath, heart palpitations, and nausea were heart related.

I had a chance to chat with my heart sister, Judy Barkley, from the WomenHeart symposium in the summer of 2020. I reached out to Judy to talk about her heart journey. I was completely taken aback when she shared, "I was recently stented for 80% blockage." My call was about her stent placement from *six years* before. Judy explained, "I had an appointment with a new cardiologist in a few days. Before the appointment I began to feel discomfort, labored breathing, and chest pain. I called my daughter who picked me up and drove to the nearest hospital. During this time the Coronavirus pandemic was in full swing, so I was left alone at the hospital. I had a cardiac workup including blood tests, echocardiogram, and chest x-rays. The attending ER doctor just happened to be my new cardiologist who I was scheduled to see in a few days. He was pleased to share that all of my tests were negative, and I was free to go home. I told him, 'No.' My doctor was confused...'No? I said, 'I'm not going home to die.' My doctor and I went back and forth, and he finally arranged for an angiogram the next day. There was 80% blockage in the same artery as six years before." Judy was an advocate for herself. She insisted the doctor look further and perform an angiogram. The doctor eventually told her, "I wish more of my patients were like you."

A 2018 study published in the *Proceedings of the National Academy of Sciences of the United States of America* found that one in every sixty-six women who has a heart attack will die in the emergency department if she is treated by a male doctor instead of a female doctor. [36] This doesn't mean that male cardiologists are less qualified than female cardiologists. It means that we have to do better and more when it comes to educating health professionals and women about heart disease and how it shows up differently in men versus in women.

Another heart sister, Brooke Tately, was in her gynecologist office a year after she suffered a heart attack. Brooke said, "Before I had a heart attack, I always thought breast cancer was the leading cause of death in women. I wanted to know why my

--------------------
[36] *"Women Die More from Heart Attacks than Men—Unless the ER Doc is Female." (2018, August 6). Retrieved from https://www.scientificamerican.com/article/women-die-more-from-heart-attacks-than-men-mdash-unless-the-er-doc-is-female/*

gynecologist never mentioned heart disease." Brooke was an advocate for other women who would come in for their gynecology appointment with the doctor.

When you're involved in your own health advocacy, you will gain a greater sense of control, increased confidence in your medical decisions, an aptitude in medical literacy, and better health outcomes.

**Here are ways to advocate for yourself:**

» Make sure you understand health insurance and specifically your policy. When you know how insurance works, you are able to traverse the health care system including reviewing medical bills for duplication and over charges.

» Plan ahead to ask questions. Doctors are usually pretty busy. Your appointment is not just a time for your doctor to do all of the talking. You should prepare your questions in advance, and use this as an opportunity to forge your doctor/patient relationship.

» Keep track of your own records. This has become incredibly easier with electronic records. The Privacy Rule of the federal Health Insurance Portability and Accountability Act (HIPAA) entitles patients to have access to their medical records.

» Analyze your medical bills. I can tell you from experience as a bodily injury adjuster, I have reviewed many medical bills and a lot have mistakes. An estimated eight out of ten medical bills have errors. Even if your medical insurance is picking up a portion or all of it—review bills for accuracy.

» Know when to get a second opinion. According to the Agency for Healthcare Research and Quality, one in twenty Americans fall victim to outpatient errors in diagnosis. Getting a second opinion could save you from unnecessary costs.

# CHAPTER SIXTEEN

# PROTECTING
# YOUR LOVED ONES

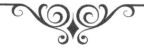

## Understanding Insurance

*"You don't buy life insurance because you are going to die but because those you love are going to live."*
*—Unknown*

I know we don't like to talk about what life would have looked like if we had not survived our heart attack or heart event. I was in insurance for so many years, I would be remiss not to have a chapter on financial and end-of-life conversations.

I conducted life insurance presentations. It is by far one of the most fulfilling jobs I've ever held. We would go to various work places, give a presentation, and offer a supplemental whole life policy for the employee and their dependents. Supplemental insurance can cover some out-of-pocket expenses—such as copayments, coinsurance, and deductible— that primary health insurance plans don't pay. Supplemental insurance policies may pay out either periodic benefits (daily or weekly) or a lump sum to the policyholder that can be used to pay for lost wages, transportation, medication, or anything else resulting from an injury or illness.

At the time of the heart attack, I worked for a company that didn't have the best benefits. They didn't have a short-term disability option, only long-term. This led me to purchase a *Critical Illness* policy. I remembered that I had purchased the policy in the wee hours of the morning right after I got out of the hospital. I called the office the next day, and sure enough I had the policy. The Critical Illness policy (sometimes called catastrophic illness insurance) pays a lump sum (you choose) directly to you when you have a catastrophic illness like cancer, heart attack, or stroke. The increments are $5,000, $10,000, $15,000, and $25,000. There is paperwork to complete...you can't just say, "I had a heart attack" and they send you a check.

As long as it wasn't a pre-existing condition, the claim will be paid.

*Hospital Indemnity* is another important insurance. Remember the passing out episodes I told you about? Some of those landed me in the hospital. A hospital indemnity policy pays you an amount of money for each day you are hospitalized. The typical amount is $500 per overnight in the hospital. In 2019 I was hospitalized unexpectedly for five days and then another night. These policies come in handy when you haven't met your deductible or need to have a procedure that requires an upfront payment.

*Life Insurance*. I know it's hard and/or very expensive to get life insurance after you have a heart attack. Don't be dismayed. You can still get coverage, and you don't have to wait five years. If you work, your employer will likely cover you, and you have to be employed with that company at your death. If you're offered a supplemental life insurance policy, get what you can without having to answer medical questions. The medical questions always include "Have you had a heart attack in the last five years?" Having a heart attack in the last five years doesn't eliminate you from qualifying for life insurance. The insurance company will make their decision to cover you based on your age, the severity of your heart event (how much blockage, how many arteries), and how much damage did your heart sustain.

My father was always very savvy when it came to finances and insurance (or least that's what we thought). It was May of 2000 when my father got sick and had the *if something happens to me* conversation with my brother Carl and me. He revealed that he was "covered." Shame on me—I was knee deep in insurance at the time...claims, but still insurance. Although I lived and breathed all things insurance, I never asked him what exactly he meant by "Everything is taken care of." Nor did I ask him where to find said paperwork documenting that everything was taken care of.

On November 9, 2001 my father was admitted to the hospital in a coma. Dad had been in the hospital three days when the doctors first conversed with my brother and me about taking him off the ventilator. We hoped he would get better. Before, we knew it my father had been in the hospital thirty days, and he hadn't made any movements on his own without the machine. I sent Carl to his apartment to find the documents. He emerged with an insurance policy for $25,000. Unfortunately, it was an *Accidental Death and Dismemberment* policy. It was of no good to us. We took my father off the ventilator on December 26, 2001. He died a few hours later. His funeral cost was paid out pocket.

These financial and end-of-life conversations can be tough to have, but they are necessary. If you have policies, let your beneficiaries know where to find everything. If you get a new policy, share with them the particulars of the policy. Tell them numbers and people to call. If you work, someone will need to call your place of employment to let them know you had a heart attack or died. Set up a call tree for the person handling your illness or death. Doing this makes their difficult role much easier.

Handling medical expenses and insurance can feel overwhelming, but take it a step at a time. When you get the hospital bill, open it gently and don't be alarmed. My bill was in excess of $30,000 for the heart attack and more when I was hospitalized and got the pacemaker. You may be thinking, "This will surely meet my deductible/maximum out of pocket." Yes, it will. However, if this is your first big medical expense, you still have to meet the deductible/out of pocket. Ask for financial assistance. Wait and see what insurance is going to pay. Ask if the hospital has any programs. If they do, enroll and keep to the payment schedule. Be honest and tell them what you can afford. This is new for you—specialty copays, medications, etc.

At the writing of this, the Affordable Care Act is still in place. It makes it so much easier to manage a chronic illness like heart disease. If you buy health insurance through your state's Marketplace, on the individual market, or through an employer with fifty or fewer employees, your plan must cover certain essential health benefits. You may need some of these services as a heart patient such as:

» Outpatient services, such as visits to your primary care physician, heart specialists, and lab tests.
» Counseling for diet, smoking cessation, alcohol abuse, or depression to learn how to lower your chance of complications from heart disease.
» Prescription drug coverage.
» Emergency room and hospital coverage.
» Rehabilitation services.

Each state determines the details of exactly what must be covered under these categories. Individual health plans may add to those minimum requirements. Before you enroll, read the plan's summary of benefits to see what specific services you'll have access to and what your costs will be. Medicare includes the essential health benefits. Both Medicare and Medicaid offer special programs for monitoring your blood pressure and other heart risks.

The Affordable Care Act has rules about the most you have to pay out-of-pocket for your medical care:

» Health plans cannot impose annual or lifetime dollar limits on your benefits.

» Your out-of-pocket costs will be limited. Health plans will have what is called an out-of-pocket maximum. Once you reach that amount through your deductibles and other copays, your insurance company covers the rest of your costs. That includes what you spend on copays and deductibles for medical services and prescriptions. The out-of-pocket maximum does not include your monthly premiums.

» You might be able to get financial help to pay for some costs if you're buying insurance through your state's Marketplace. Check with your accountant regarding a tax credit to lower your insurance premiums.

» You may qualify for Medicaid coverage, even if you haven't in the past. This will depend on how much you earn and the state you live in.

# CHAPTER SEVENTEEN

# THE FENCE POST

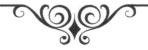

## *Focus on You!*

*"The tragedies that define our lives, they are the fence post on which the rest of our lives hang."*
—Beth Pearson, This is Us Season 5 Premiere

I was watching one of my favorite shows, *This is Us*, as I worked on my final thoughts for this book. It was the two-hour premiere of season five. Beth is having a conversation with her husband Randall. He is down about a lot of things. What she says to him inspired me to deeply reflect on my life. *"The tragedies that define our lives, they are the fence post on which the rest of our lives hang."*

Life is comprised of many defining moments, both tragedies and blessings. Sometimes what initially seems like a tragedy can turn out to be a blessing. Have you experienced that? I remember graduating from high school, college, and graduate school. I'll never forget my first house. It was a 3-bedroom, 2-bath, 2-car garage home with brick on the front. I had to do work equity (that's code for paint the walls yourself). I was twenty-five and didn't care because I had purchased a built-just-for-me house. I have many good memories of the celebration of my wedding day, even though we divorced seven years later. I choose to focus more on the blessing than the tragedy. I loved my grandparents dearly, and they lived with us the last few years of their life. They passed away within a year of each other, I was heartbroken, and old enough to understand life and death.

When my good friend Tammy passed, it was a defining moment. We were both forty-eight years old. She was diagnosed with breast cancer and did everything right to embrace a host of "preventative" measures—yet the cancer found its way to so many places in her body. I was almost two years post heart attack, and it became very clear to me that we are all given an unknown specified period of time to make an impact, or not, with our life. The choice of the type of legacy we leave is ours.

Another of my defining moments is I started Customized Learning, Inc., an insurance pre-licensing school. I was the first African American person to create such a business in Indiana. Starting, growing, and maintaining that business was very fulfilling as I saw the people who attended pursue their goals, and I made an impact with my life.

I hope my moments have stirred up memories for you of those events that define your life. Fighting an illness or surviving a heart attack is part of the defining moments conversation. You decide what your fence post looks like.

After the heart attack when Mom and I finally got to the two-bedroom bungalow, there were times I would venture outside, hold my face up to the sun, and just sit and think. I was full of gratitude. I wanted to be about the business of showing God just how grateful I was for sparing my life. Not even two months post heart event, I wanted to help someone. I tried to volunteer for the American Heart Association, but it was too soon for me and fortunately didn't work out.

When Mom and I arrived back in Dallas after my initial time of recovery, we hadn't been home five minutes when Karen and Dottie from our church arrived with bags of groceries filled with heart healthy foods. There was salmon, chicken breast, turkey, shrimp, tilapia, and every fresh vegetable and fruit you can think of. We both were so grateful. Through my tears I managed to ask, "How can we ever thank you for all of this?" They both looked from Mom to me and Karen said, "Just do it for someone else." That was in August 2015.

For the longest time I couldn't figure out how to do it for someone else. At the time I was a Girl Scout leader. I decided to make sure my troop knew how to perform CPR and the steps to take in an emergency. The girls were pretty young when we went through the class, and it was a good experience and valuable lesson.

I did a few more projects over the next two years, but I felt like something was still missing in the impact I wanted to make. I called it "my warm fuzzy feeling" of being able to say, "I'm making a difference, God. Thank you for sparing my life, and I'm paying it forward."

Then one sunny afternoon during a walk, it came to me. Together Karen and Dottie helped to give my heart the fresh start it needed. I could too and finally be able to "do it for someone else." I started a 501(c)3 dedicated to giving hearts a fresh start. It's simply called *Fresh Start for Your Heart*. https://www.freshstartheart.org. We are the only non-profit who will send a grocery delivery of heart healthy foods to heart event survivors. It's a young organization, and it's part of my fencepost.

I also started Any Day CPR Training. https://www.anydaycpr.com. I teach people—and teach people to teach people—what to do in an emergency. They learn how to physically pump blood to the heart and brain if a victim is in cardiac arrest. Please give yourself, and others you know, the priceless gift of CPR. The life you save could be your own or someone you love.

My fence post is full. On July 2, 2020 I celebrated my five-year heart-aversary. I started a podcast—**Healing Hope for Your Heart**. The purpose is to share heart stories as messages of prevention, early detection, accurate diagnosis, and overall heart disease awareness. Our goal is to eradicate heart disease one heart story at a time.

If you've read this book just a couple of months into your recovery, focus on yourself and getting better. Self-care isn't selfish, it's necessary for a healthy life. When you're feeling stronger, please let me know your thoughts about this book and your heart story. I would love to hear from you.

# CHAPTER EIGHTEEN
# ONE LAST REFLECTION

## Lessons from a Heart Attack Survivor

*"These life lessons...I assure you haven't been lost on me."*
—Denise Castille

Heart disease is the leading cause of death in the United States for both men and women. Every minute someone dies from a heart disease related event. While one in thirty-one American women dies from breast cancer each year, heart disease is the cause of one out of every three deaths. Heart disease affects women of all ages. Sixty-four percent of women who die suddenly of coronary heart disease had no previous symptoms.

Five years ago, on July 2, 2015, I had a medical emergency when a clot formed and blocked blood flow to my heart causing what cardiologists know as the "widow-maker" heart attack. A heart attack is plausibly one of the most tragic and unexpected events you will experience. It is life altering.

This health scare helped me to prioritize my life, and it taught me five incredible lessons.

1. **Take the cup by the handle**. This is one of the many sayings I grew up hearing from my mom. It meant make it happen...do it. Post heart attack it meant following doctor's orders to take medications as prescribed, participate in cardiac rehabilitation, and manage the risks for heart disease—every day as though my life depends on it. Live up to your full potential. See situations the way they are, not how you think they should be, and make it happen.

2. **Triumph or Tragedy...You decide the trajectory**. There is an entire chapter in this book on the myriad of emotions you go through following a heart attack. We can either use the experience as a wake-up call— leave a stressful job, lose weight, stop smoking, and eat healthier—or we can slump into a *woe is me* mentality and miss the opportunity to become a better version of ourselves.

3. **Every day is a mulligan.** My brother, Carl, who is not a golfer, told me about this term and its meaning. "A mulligan is when a golfer hits a bad shot and is given a chance to do it over again." Laying on the floor waiting for paramedics to arrive, *I asked God not to let me die like this.* God blessed me with a mulligan. A chance to have more time with my family and friends, laugh more, and make a difference.

4. **Life is short.** No matter how many mulligans we get, life is still short. Prior to the heart attack I was busy—too busy to look after my health. Don't be so consumed and busy with the present you lose sight of the future.

5. **Still here for a purpose.** I asked God to not let me die like this—and He didn't. But not because I asked. I'm sure people bargain with God all the time. I survived on July 2, 2015 because there is still purpose in my life. I truly believe that when our purpose is fulfilled, our time here is done. Your survival means you have purpose.

Have you ever looked around and wondered, "How did I get here?" For me it was gradually, one sign and symptom at a time:

» **Extreme exhaustion**. You may suddenly feel fatigued or winded after doing something you had no problem doing in the past.

» **Throat or jaw pain**. On their own, throat or jaw pain isn't heart related. If there is chest pain that spreads up to the throat or jaw, it could indicate a heart attack.

» **Dizzy or lightheaded**. Lots of things can cause you to feel dizzy or lightheaded. Not drinking enough water, or eating enough, or standing up too quickly. If you're unsteady/wobbly and you have chest pain, call or have someone call 911.

» **Pain that spreads to the arm**. This is a classic heart attack symptom—pain radiates down the left side of the body.

» **Sweating**. Breaking out in a cold sweat for no apparent reason is a heart attack sign.

» **Legs, ankles, and feet are swollen**. This is a sign that your heart isn't pumping blood as effectively as it should. When the heart doesn't pump fast enough, it causes the blood to back up in the veins and causes bloating.

» **Irregular heartbeats**. When you're excited or startled, your heart may beat faster than usual. If your heart is beating fast often, or rapidly for more than a few seconds, this is an important detail for the doctor.

» **Nagging cough.** Typically, a cough is not a heart disease indicator; however, if you have heart disease or you're at risk, you should pay attention to a cough that produces white or pink mucus and stays around. This could be a sign of heart failure. When the heart can't keep up with your body's demands, it causes blood to leak back into the lungs.

Stay alert and aware of the gradually. Everything we do or don't do has a consequence. *Gradually* may one day become *suddenly*!

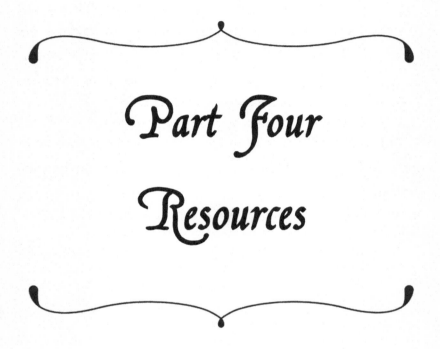

# Part Four

# Resources

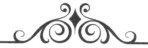

# HEART ATTACK AND SUDDEN CARDIAC ARREST HOW THEY ARE DIFFERENT

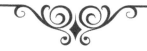

## *When and How to Use CPR*

As a CPR training business owner and instructor, <u>www. anydaycpr.com</u>, I would be remiss if I didn't share with you the differences between a heart attack and sudden cardiac arrest. The two are often used interchangeably, but they are not the same. A *heart attack* happens when the blood flow to the heart is blocked, and *sudden cardiac arrest* occurs when the heart malfunctions and suddenly stops beating. They are often explained as a heart attack involves circulation and sudden cardiac arrest is an electrical issue.

Heart attacks may be immediate and severe, but the symptoms can be present for days, weeks, or even months. During a heart attack, the heart doesn't stop beating; however, a heart attack can lead to cardiac arrest. Call 911 for a paramedic and ambulance. CPR is not needed in a heart attack situation unless cardiac arrest occurs.

Sudden cardiac arrest happens without warning. It is triggered by an electrical malfunction that causes the heart to have an irregular heartbeat (arrhythmia). When this occurs the heart *ceases to pump blood* to the brain, lungs, and other organs. Within a very short period of time (seconds, not minutes), the person loses consciousness and has no pulse. Death occurs within minutes if the victim does not receive help.

When sudden cardiac arrest happens, call 911 for a paramedic and begin cardiopulmonary resuscitation (CPR) immediately to keep the blood flowing. Here are the CPR steps:

>> Ensure your surroundings are safe. You won't be any good to the victim if you get hurt.
>> Tap and shout. Tap on the shoulders of the adult or child and shout, "Are you okay, are you okay?"
>> Shout for help. Ask someone to call 911, and get an Automated External Defibrillator (AED). When the AED arrives, use it immediately. The AED has a built-

in mechanism to guide you through each step with voice commands.

» Check for breathing by scanning the chest for five to ten seconds. See if the chest rises.

» If the victim is **not breathing,** begin chest compressions. If the victim is breathing but unresponsive place them in the recovery position (turn them on their left side) and wait until emergency help arrives.

» Kneeling next to the victim, place the heel of your hand in the center of the chest on the breastbone. Position hands between the nipples.

» Place the other hand directly on top of the first.

» Interlace your fingers.

» Keep your arms straight.

» Push straight down at a depth of two inches; provide compressions at a rate of 100 per minute (allow the chest to recoil; do not lift your hands off the chest).

» After giving thirty compressions: give two quick breaths. Continue with cycles of 30 compressions and 2 rescue breaths until they recover, or emergency help arrives.

# Recommended Reading

## Books

Back to Life After a Heart Crisis: A Doctor and His Wife Share Their 8 Step Cardiac Comeback *Plan*, Marc Wallack, M.D and Jamie Colby with Alisa Bowman. The Penguin Group (2010)

Best Practices for a Healthy Heart-How to Stop Heart Disease Before or After It Starts, Sarah Samaan, MD. The Experiment Publishing (2011)

*Heart Health for Black Women,* Dr. Beverly Yates. Marlow and Company Publishing (2000)

*How Doctors Think*, Jerome Groopman, M.D. Mariner Books Publishing (2008)

*Know Your Real Risk of a Heart Attack,* Dr. Warrick Bishop. Published by Dr. Warrick Bishop (2018)

Optimize Your Heart: A Practical Guide to Lowering Your Risk of a Heart Attack or Stroke, Andy Beal, CPT. Andy Beal/Marketing Pilgrim, LLC (2020)

The Amazing Way to Reverse Heart Disease Naturally, Eric R. Braverman, M.D. and Dasha Braverman, B.S., R.P.A-C. Basic Health Publications (2004)

The Cancer Survivor's Companion: Practical Ways to Cope with Your Feelings after Cancer. Lucy Atkins and Dr. Francis Goodhart. Piatkus Publishing (2013)

The Cardiac Recovery Handbook: The Complete Guide to Life After a Heart Attack or Heart

*Surgery,* 2nd Edition, Paul Kligfield, M.D. (Author), Michelle D. Seaton (Author), Frederic Flach, MD KCHS (Afterword). Hatherleigh Press (2006)

The End of Heart Disease: The Eat to Live Plan to Prevent and Reverse Heart Disease (Eat for *Life),* Joel Fuhrman, M.D. Harper One An Imprint of Harper Collins Publisher (2016)

The Smart Woman's Guide to Heart Health: Dr. Sarah's Seven Steps to a Heart Loving Lifestyle, Sarah Samaan MD. Brown Books Publishing Group (2009)

# Blogs/Journals/Magazines

**EatingWell Magazine**
Website Address: http://www.eatingwell.com/

**Heart Advisor Magazine**
Website Address: https://www.heart-advisor.com/

**Healthy A Lifestyle Magazine**
Website Address: http://healthymagazine.com/the-guide-to-a-healthy-heart/

**Heart Healthy Living**
Website Address:
https://www.discountmags.com/magazine/heart-healthy-living

**Prevention**
Website Address: https://www.prevention.com/

**Self Magazine**
Website Address: www.self.com

**Shape Magazine**

Website Address: www.shape.com

# PODCASTS

- » American Heart Association
- » At the Heart
- » Healing Hope for Your Heart
- » Heart Doc VIP
- » The Healthy Heart Show
- » The Heart Healthy Hustle

# GENERAL INFORMATION

## American Association of Retired Persons (AARP)

601 East Street, NW

Washington DC 20049

Toll-Free Nationwide: 1-888-OUR-AARP (1-888-687-2277)

Toll-Free Spanish: 1-877-342-2277

Web Address: www.aarp.org

## The American Diabetes Association

800-342-2283

Arlington County, VA

Web Address: www.diabetes.org

The American Diabetes Association is a United States-based nonprofit that seeks to educate the public about diabetes and to help those affected by it through funding research to manage, cure, and prevent diabetes.

## American Heart Association

National Center

7272 Greenville Avenue

Dallas, TX 75231

1-800-AHA-USA-1 or 1-800-242-8721 or Outside US: +1 (214) 570-5978

Web Address: www.heart.org/

The American Heart Association is a nonprofit organization in the United States that funds cardiovascular medical research, educates consumers on healthy living, and fosters appropriate cardiac care in an effort to reduce disability and deaths caused by cardiovascular disease and stroke.

## American Stroke Association

National Center

7272 Greenville Avenue

Dallas TX 75231

1-888-4-STROKE or 1-888-478-7653

Web Address: www.stroke.org/

The American Stroke Association is a relentless force for a healthier world with fewer strokes. They team up with millions of volunteers to prevent, treat and beat stroke by funding innovative research, fighting for stronger public health policies, and providing lifesaving tools and information.

## Association of Black Cardiologists

122 East 42nd Street

18th Floor

New York, NY 10168

800-753-9222

Web Address: www.abcardio.org

The Association of Black Cardiologists is an organization founded to bring special attention to the adverse impact of cardiovascular disease on African Americans.

## Black Heart Association

1029 Kaylie Street

Grand Prairie, TX 75052

817-683-8869

Website Address: https://blackheartassociation.org/

Black Heart Association is at the forefront of research, prevention, treatment, and education surrounding heart disease in the Black community.

## Fresh Start for Your Heart

P.O. Box 6487

McKinney, TX 75069

972-589-6820

Email: info@freshstartheart.org

Web Address: http://www.freshstartheart.org

Fresh Start for Your Heart is a Texas based nonprofit organization brings awareness to heart disease through programming and podcast. The organization provides a one-time heart healthy grocery delivery to women who have suffered a heart event.

## Heart Healthy Women

Web Address: hearthealthywomen.org

Provides information for patients, providers, and caregivers regarding the diagnosis and treatment of heart disease in women.

## Medscape

Web Address: https://www.medscape.com/

Provide the latest research on a variety of medical topics, including heart disease. Sign up to receive newsletters from them.

## The Mended Hearts, Inc.

7272 Greenville Avenue

Dallas, TX 75231-4596

888-HEART99 or 888-432-7899

Email: info@mendedhearts.org

Web Address: http://mendedhearts.org

Mended Hearts offer support groups nationally to patients who have had a heart event, and they can make referrals to a support groups in your area.

## Office on Women's Health

U.S. Department of Health and Human Services

200 Independence Avenue, SW Room 712E

Washington, DC 20201

1-800-994-9662

Web Address: womenshealth.gov

A federal government site providing information and resources on women's health topics including heart disease.

## Society of Women's Health Research

1025 Connecticut Avenue NW

Suite 1104

Washington, DC 20036

202-223-8224

Web Address: swhr.org

General Inquiries: info@swhr.org

Partnerships, Policy Council Membership, and Philanthropy: development@swhr.org

Policy and Advocacy: policy@swhr.org

Science: science@swhr.org

Media Inquiries: communications@swhr.org

The Society for Women's Health Research (SWHR) promotes research on biological sex differences in disease and improving women's health through science, policy, and education.

**The Heart Truth**
National Heart, Lung, and Blood Institute
Building 31
Bethesda, MD. 20892
Web Address: https://www.nhlbi.nih.gov/health-topics/education-and-awareness/heart-truth
Provide education and awareness campaign information for women.

**WebMD**
Web Address: www.Webmd.com
A source for information and news regarding a multitude of diseases and health issues including heart disease. Sign up for their free newsletter.

**WomenHeart: The National Coalition of Women and Heart Disease**
1100 17th St NW #500
Washington, DC 20036
202-728-7199
Email: mail@womenheart.org
Web Address: www.womenheart.org
Provide information, resources, and support for women living with heart disease.

# INSURANCE

**Healthcare.gov**

Website Address: https://www.healthcare.gov/how-can-i-get-consumer-help-if-i-have-insurance/

Phone: 800-318-2596 (TTY: 855-889-4325)

Provides answers to questions about health coverage.

**Medicare.Gov**

Website Address: https://www.medicare.gov/contacts/

Everything about Medicare including what's covered, drug coverage, claims and appeals, managing your health, and forms

**National Association of Insurance Commissioners (NAIC)**

Website Address: https://content.naic.org/consumer.htm

Helps consumers navigate insurance and make better decisions.

**Patient Advocate Foundation (PAF)**

Website Address: https://www.patientadvocate.org/explore-our-resources/interacting-with-your-insurer/what-do-i-do-if-i-cant-get-answers-from-my-insurance-company/

Contact PAF when you have questions for your insurance company that go unanswered.

**USA GOV**

Website Address: https://www.usa.gov/finding-health-insurance

Provides information regarding Affordable Care Act, Continuation of Coverage (COBRA), Health Plans, Long Term Care and Health Insurance, and Health Resources for People with Disabilities

# MEDICATION MANAGEMENT

**Paying for Senior Care**

(206) 462-5728

Web Address: https://www.payingforseniorcare.com

This organization provides educational information. They help find or choose a local assisted living community, in-home care agency, or other senior care provider. Additionally, they may be able to provide financial resources.

**Cureatr**

Phone: 646-661-5168

Web Address: https://www.cureatr.com

Cureatr is a comprehensive medication management (CMM) solutions company providing real-time, universal access to accurate medication data. They help health plans, healthcare organizations, and patients make sure medications are taken appropriately, effectively, and most of all safely.

## GoodRx

233 Wilshire Blvd.

Suite #990

Santa Monica, CA

Phone: 855-268-2822

GoodRx is an American healthcare company that operates a telemedicine platform and a free-to-use website and mobile app that track prescription drug prices in the United States and provide free drug coupons for discounts on medications. GoodRx checks more than 75,000 pharmacies in the United States.

## RxList

Web Address: http://www.rxlist.com

On RxList information on medications can be found using the Drugs A - Z list (an alphabetical listing of both brand and generic drug names) or by entering the generic or brand drug name in the search box at the top of the page and clicking search. If you need to identify a pill, you can use their pill identification tool.

## Rx.com

Web Address: http://www.rx.com

An online pharmacy.

# MEDICAL RECORDS MANAGEMENT

**Health IT.gov**

https://www.healthit.gov/topic/patient-access-information-individuals-get-it-check-it-use-it

The Office of the National Coordinator for Health Information Technology

https://www.healthit.gov/how-to-get-your-health-record/

# MENTAL HEALTH

**American Psychological Association**

750 First Street, NE

Washington, DC 20002-4242

(800) 374-2721 or (202) 336-5500

Web Address: www.apa.org

American Psychological Association provides clinical psychologist referrals.

**American Psychiatric Association**

800 Maine Ave, SW

Washington, D.C.

888-35-PSYCH or 888-357-7924

Web Address: www.psych.org

American Psychiatric Association provides referrals to psychiatrist in your area.

**Anxiety Disorders Association of America (ADAA)**

8701 Georgia Avenue

Suite #412

Silver Spring, MD. 20910

240-485-1001

Web Address: https://adaa.org/

**Better Help**

990 Villa Street

Mountain View, CA 94041

Web Address: www.betterhelp.com/

Better Help provides online grief counseling covering depression, stress, anxiety, and other topics.

**National Mental Health Consumers' Self-Help Clearing House (NMHCSH)**

1211 Chestnut St., Suite 1100

Philadelphia, PA 19107

(800) 553-4539 or (215) 751-1810

Web Address: https://www.mhselfhelp.org/

Email: info@mhselfhelp.org

National Mental Health Consumers' Self-Help Clearing House is a large portal to help with finding self-help groups in your area.

**Sondermind**

844-256-9902

Web Address: https://www.sondermind.com/client-and-therapist-customer-support

Sondermind connects you with a licensed therapist via video telehealth or in person sessions (accepted by most insurance carriers).

**Talk Space Grief Counseling**

(800) 273-8255

Web Address: https://www.talkspace.com/

Talk Space connects you with a licensed therapist. May be available through most Employer Assistance Programs (EAP).

# NUTRITION/EXERCISE

**American Heart Association**

National Center

7272 Greenville Avenue

Dallas, TX 75231

1-800-AHA-USA-1 or 1-800-242-8721 or Outside US: +1 (214) 570-5978

Web Address: www.heart.org/

## American Society for Nutrition – Nutrition Research and Science

Web Address: https://www.nutrition.org

Provides nutrition-based information.

## Calorie Control Council

Web Address: https://www.caloriecontrol.org

An international organization providing information for cutting calories and fat in your diet, achieving and maintaining a healthy weight.

# CALORIE COUNTING APPS AND WEBSITES

## MyFitnessPal

Tracks your weight and calculates a recommended daily intake. There is also an exercise and food log.

## Lose It!

A health tracker that includes an easy-to-use food diary and exercise log. There is also a way to connect the pedometer to other fitness devices. Based on your height, weight, and goals, Lose It! provides personalized recommendations for calorie intake.

## FatSecret
This is a free calorie counter. It includes a food diary, nutrition database, healthy recipes, exercise log, weight chart, and journal. There is a built in barcode scanner to help you track packaged foods.

## Cron-o-meter
This app lets you easily keep track of what you eat, exercises, and body weight.

# NATIONWIDE FITNESS CENTERS

- » UFC Gym
- » Fitness Body Boot Camp
- » Gold's Gym
- » Anytime Fitness
- » Snap Fitness 24/7
- » Gym Guyz
- » Cycle Bar
- » World Gym
- » Workout Anytime 24/7
- » 9Round
- » Orange Theory Fitness
- » LA Fitness

# Acknowledgements

I'm incredibly humbled and appreciative...first and foremost for, Shirley Castille, my encourager cheerleader/mom, who brought me endless cups of tea, wouldn't let me give up and got me, quickly, back on track when I was derailed. Thank you for believing I could write a book.

Heartfelt thanks to my only sibling, Carl Castille, for insightful feedback, encouragement and love.

A special and gracious thank you to Marie Bianco, Farmington Hills Michigan Fire Department Paramedics: Stephen, Kevin and Nick, Botsford Memorial Hospital Emergency Room team, and Dr. Mark Rasak. If not for each one of you—I wouldn't be here to write this book. Thank you for taking care of me.

My favorite uncle, Rev. James Bailey, Jr. and his wife, Anna Bailey (who is also a heart attack survivor) I am so grateful for your support and willingness to help bring this book to fruition. Every heart sister (and brother) who have shared their story with me—Catherine Paour, Kelsey Taryn, Scott Decker, Lisa Ballow, Sharvonne Williams, Jeen Beverly, Jerome Spearman,

Cynthia Walker, Missallen Sheila, Rachel Hobart on behalf of my youngest heart brother, baby Dean, the entire WomenHeart Champion Class of 2017 ---- each of you are an inspiration and I am thankful that you are here to share your journey.

For as long as I can remember I have wanted to write a book. If not for Joan T. Randall's 30-day writing challenge this book would have stayed a dream. Thank you, Joan and your publishing team, for coming along side and helping me bring my dream to life. I am eternally grateful.

I am forever beholden to hands down the best editor, ever, Patty Lauterjung. She pushed me beyond what I thought my limits were and helped me to tell my story in a way that is authentically me.

I have a heart of gratitude for Distinguished Toastmaster, Mj Presley, for planting the seed about writing a book about my HEART journey.

I am thankful for Addison Hoyt Williams for your passion as a photographer and capturing the essence of me for my book cover.

# About the Author

Denise Castille was born and raised in Indianapolis, Indiana. She has a Master of Business Administration from University of Indianapolis and a Master of Human Resource Management. Denise attended Tuskegee University for undergraduate studies.

She is the founder and executive director of Fresh Start for Your Heart, a 501(c)3 nonprofit. An organization Denise founded to pay it forward for other heart event survivors. She is the CEO of Any Day CPR Training, LLC. Denise is a proud member of Delta Sigma Theta Sorority, Inc. She is an active member of District 50 Toastmasters. She holds a Distinguished Toastmaster designation from Toastmasters International.

Denise has one sibling, Carl Castille, Sr. She has three nephews—Christopher Castille, Carl Jr. Castille and Ethan Rodman. One beautiful niece, Chloe, who she gets to tutor virtually.

Denise loves to travel. She and mom have been on 20+ cruises to date. She is a voracious reader. She loves to laugh and next on Denise's bucket list is doing something in the comedy realm.  She is active in her church, Grace Church, as a children's church teacher.

Denise lives in McKinney, TX with her mom, Miss Shirley.

Made in USA - Kendallville, IN
1236790_9781952756191
02.19.2021 0842